T0298544

Children's Services:
Social Policy, Research, and Practice

Volume 5, Number 1, 2002

**Special Issue: Evaluating Systems of Care: The Comprehensive
Community Mental Health Services for Children and
Their Families Program
Guest Editors: E. Wayne Holden and Ana Maria Brannan**

CHILDREN'S SERVICES: SOCIAL POLICY, RESEARCH, AND PRACTICE, 5(1), 1

Background for the Special Issue

E. Wayne Holden and Ana Maria Brannan
ORC Macro
Atlanta, GA

This issue of *Children's Services: Social Policy, Research, and Practice* consists of five articles profiling different aspects of the national evaluation of the Comprehensive Community Mental Health Services for Children and Their Families Program, sponsored by the Center for Mental Health Services within the Substance Abuse and Mental Health Services Administration. Over the last 8 years, this program has provided grants to 67 communities across the United States to develop community-based systems of care for children with serious emotional disturbance and their families. A comprehensive, multilevel evaluation has been conducted that has provided information to local grantee communities and the federal government on the implementation and effectiveness of systems of care. Many individuals across the country have been involved in this effort, including the children and families participating in the evaluation, evaluation and program staff in the funded communities, advocacy groups, other collaborators in universities and other private and public organizations, personnel from the Center for Mental Health Services, and national evaluation staff members. The collaborative efforts of all of these groups under the leadership of the Child, Adolescent and Family Branch at the Center for Mental Health Services have made this large-scale program evaluation a reality. The articles included in this issue touch on a range of questions that the evaluation is designed to address and provide more general information on the system-of-care approach to addressing children's mental health problems.

This special issue could not have been completed successfully without the support provided by Leza Young, a research associate at ORC Macro who provides administrative support to the national evaluation. Her organizational skills, proofreading, and editing were instrumental in completing each of the articles included in this issue.

CHILDREN'S SERVICES: SOCIAL POLICY, RESEARCH, AND PRACTICE, 5(1), 3–20

Overview of the National Evaluation of the Comprehensive Community Mental Health Services for Children and Their Families Program and Summary of Current Findings

Brigitte Manteuffel and Robert L. Stephens
ORC Macro
Atlanta, GA

Rolando Santiago
Center for Mental Health Services
Substance Abuse and Mental Health Services Administration
Washington, DC

In this article we present an overview of descriptive and longitudinal outcome data collected by the national evaluation of the Comprehensive Community Mental Health for Children and Their Families Program. This program, supported by the federal Center for Mental Health Services at the Substance Abuse Mental Health Services Administration, has established systems of care for mental health services in 67 communities throughout the United States. Among the 22 communities receiving grants in 1993 and 1994, descriptive information was collected on 44,640 children who received services. Longitudinal outcome study enrollment included 18,884 children, with data collected on 2,580 children who continued in services through 24 months. The average age of children served was 12.1 years; 61.9% were boys, 54.7% were White, and 60.3% had annual household incomes below $15,000. Primary diagnoses included conduct-related disorders (29.3%), attention deficit hyperactivity disorder (13.6%), and depression or dysthymia (26%). Changes in children's behaviors and functioning were examined to 2 years in services; 44.6% of children exhibited clinically significant improvements in behavioral and emotional symptoms at 2 years, and 49.5% showed similar changes in functional impairment.

Requests for reprints should be sent to Brigitte Manteuffel, ORC Macro, 3 Corporate Square, Suite 370, Atlanta, GA 30329. E-mail: bmanteuf@macroint.com

The first Surgeon General's Report on Mental Health (U.S. Department of Health and Human Services, 1999) was a landmark event detailing the significant resources that have been devoted to the development of mental health services over the past several decades. The report concluded that approximately 20% or 1 in 5 children are affected at any one point in time by a mental health disorder. In 1993, an estimated 9 million to 13 million children and adolescents in the United States (14% to 20%) suffered from a mental health disorder diagnosable under the *Diagnostic and Statistical Manual of Mental Disorders* (4th ed. [*DSM–IV*]; American Psychiatric Association, 1994), and about 3.5 million children (3% to 5%) experienced serious emotional disturbance with accompanying functional impairment. Considerable progress has been made in addressing the mental health needs of children; yet children with these needs and their families continue to be underserved, and many questions remain regarding the development of effective community-based mental health services for youth. These questions span a wide range of issues including such areas as the accurate identification of children and families needing services, the integration of a wide array of interventions into community mental health services, efficient financing of services, and continuing efforts to reduce the stigma associated with mental health disorders among children and their families. As Farmer (2000) identified, understanding system level outcomes, as well as individual level outcomes experienced by children and families, is particularly challenging.

The Comprehensive Community Mental Health Services for Children and Their Families Program, administered by the federal Center for Mental Health Services within the Substance Abuse and Mental Health Services Administration, represents the largest federal investment ever to develop community-based mental health services for children and their families. This program, which began to support communities in 1993, provides grants to states, communities, territories, and Native American tribes to improve and expand their systems of care to meet the needs of children and adolescents with serious emotional disturbances and their families. In total, 67 grants have been awarded to communities in 43 states. In 1993 and 1994, 5-year grants were made to 22 communities; in 1997, 9 communities were funded; in 1998, 14 communities were funded; and in 1999 and 2000, 22 more communities were funded.

The system-of-care program theory (Stroul & Friedman, 1986) asserts that to serve children with serious emotional disturbance, service delivery systems need to offer a wide array of accessible, community-based service options that center on children's individual needs, include the family in treatment planning and delivery, and provide services in a culturally competent manner. An emphasis is placed on serving children in the least restrictive setting. In addition, because many children with serious emotional disturbance use a variety of services and have contact with several child-serving agencies, service coordination and interagency collaboration are critical. The system-of-care approach holds that if services are provided in this manner, outcomes for children and families will be better than can be achieved in traditional service delivery systems. In the system-of-care program theory model, agencies in various child-serving sectors, such as education, juvenile justice, mental health, and child welfare, work together to provide the wide array of services needed by children with serious emotional disturbance and their families. Built upon the Child and Adolescent Service System Program philosophy that calls for services to be child centered, family focused, community based, and culturally competent, the model emphasizes the need to (a) broaden the range of nonresidential community-based services, (b) strengthen case planning across child-serving sectors, and (c) increase case management capacity to ensure that services work together across sectors and providers.

NATIONAL EVALUATION

To examine the implementation of system-of-care theory, as described by the model, the national evaluation of this program was designed to answer the following overarching questions:

- To what extent do systems of care develop and improve over time?
- What services do children and families receive, what service utilization patterns do they experience, and what are the costs of those services?
- What are the characteristics of the children and families served by systems of care?
- To what extent do client outcomes improve over time?
- To what extent do children and families experience service delivery in keeping with the system-of-care program model?
- To what extent can improvements in children's behavior and functioning be associated with a system-of-care approach?

To address these research questions, a complex, multiple component design was used. Five study components comprised the core of the evaluation: (a) a collection of descriptive data about each child and family served by the program; (b) a longitudinal outcome study of a subset of children and families receiving services; (c) an assessment at the system level to examine the development of the system of care in each community over the course of the funding period; (d) an assessment of the types of services received by program participants, utilization patterns, and associated costs through examination of data recorded in management information systems; and (e) a study comparing three communities with system-of-care funding to three matched communities without funding.

Information presented here is limited to descriptive and longitudinal outcome data from communities funded in 1993 and 1994. Descriptive information including demographics and clinical or service histories provides a comprehensive picture of the characteristics of children and families served across system-of-care grant communities. The outcome study examines changes in child clinical and functional status and family life over time among those receiving system-of-care services. Collecting data in each grantee community enhances the understanding of the unique circumstances found within a particular community that may impact outcomes for children. Examining these features along with changes children and families experience as a result of receiving services in a system of care can contribute to the development of stronger programs in all communities.

METHOD

Study participants were children from birth to age 22 with serious emotional disturbances and their families receiving services supported by the Comprehensive Community Mental Health Services for Children and Their Families Program in 22 communities that received 5-year program grants in 1993 and 1994. These communities were located in 16 states, ranged from rural to urban in setting, and had diverse ethnic populations. Children participating in the study entered services between 1994 and 1999. Descriptive data were collected on any children receiving services, whereas children between ages 5 and 17.5 years at entry into services, who did not have siblings in the evaluation and had caregivers who consented to their own and their children's (for youth 11 and older) participation, were followed longitudinally in the outcome study. A caregiver was defined as the person who had primary caretaking responsibility during the assessment period.

The outcome study followed a simple pretest–posttest replacement design, with data collected at intake into services, at 6 months, 1 year, and annually thereafter up to 36 months for as long as children remained in services. The length of time children remained in the outcome study was also influenced by timing of entry into services. That is, children entering services in the second year of funding could be followed longer than children entering services in the fourth year of funding. Additional data were collected as families exited services. When children and families exited services (and therefore the evaluation), or were lost to follow-up, they were replaced with a new family entering services. The number of children enrolled in the outcome study varied across grant communities for reasons that included the size of the community and the proposed program. In total, 21 of the 22 1993–1994 grant communities participated in the outcome study; participation of one community was hindered by the large geographical area served and limited available local staff for the evaluation. Data aggregated from these communities were used in this study. Outcome study enrollment included 18,884 children; at follow-up, data were collected on 8,065 children at 6 months, 5,995 children at 12 months, 2,580 children at 24 months, and 644 children at 36 months. Given the small number of children for whom data were available at 36 months, longitudinal analyses were limited to outcomes at 24 months.

Participants

Data were obtained on at least one evaluation instrument for 44,640 children enrolled in system-of-care programs across the 22 communities. Due to missing data and variations in descriptive data collection across communities, the number of children for whom data were available varied. Among 40,322 children for whom data were available, ages ranged from less than 1 year to 23 years, with a mean of 12.1 years (SD = 4.05); 21.3% were under age 9, 42.8% were between 9 and 14 years old, and 35.9% were 15 years and older. About two thirds of the children (61.9%) were boys (N = 40,428). Slightly more than half were White (54.7%); 24.5% were Hispanic; 14.7% were African American; 3.4% were Asian, native Hawaiian, or Pacific Islander; and 1.8% were Native American or Alaskan Native (N = 38,201).

Additional descriptive information was obtained for more restricted samples. Among 9,855 children, most (47.8%) were in the custody of their biological mothers only; 25.9% were in the custody of two parents (biological or biological and step), 5.1% were in their fathers' custody, 7.1% were in the custody of guardians (e.g., adoptive parents, foster parents, aunts or uncles, grandparents), 10.3% were wards of the state, and 3.9% had some other custody arrangement. Family income data for 8,142 children indicated that 60.4% of families had annual incomes below $15,000, 18.2% had annual incomes between $15,000 and $24,999, and 21.4% had incomes of $25,000 or higher.

Measures

Descriptive data.   Child and family descriptive information included demographics, child and family risk factors, referral source, family income, custody status, mental health service use history, diagnoses, and presenting problems.

Child Behavior Checklist and Youth Self-Report.   Behavioral and emotional problems were assessed using the Child Behavior Checklist (CBCL; Achenbach, 1991a), and the Youth Self-Report (YSR; completed by children 11 years of age and older; Achenbach, 1991b), both widely used measures of children's behavioral and emotional problems in the field of children's mental health services. The CBCL consists of 118 problem behavior items classified into *internalizing* or *externalizing* behaviors. The YSR uses 112 items to assess the same behaviors from the youth's perspective. Internalizing, externalizing, and total problem T scores can be calculated, with scores above 63 falling in the clinical range.

Child and Adolescent Functional Assessment Scale.   Level of functioning was assessed using the Child and Adolescent Functional Assessment Scale

(CAFAS; Hodges, 1990). The CAFAS was designed to be used to assess the degree of psychosocial functioning of children or adolescents ranging in age from 5 to 17.5 across eight domains: (a) role performance in school, (b) role performance at home, (c) role performance in the community, (d) behavior toward others, (e) moods and emotions, (f) self-harmful behaviors, (g) substance abuse, and (h) thinking. Scores in each of these domains and a total score based on the eight subscales are calculated, with higher scores indicating greater functional impairment.

Residential Living Environments and Placement Stability Scale.   The Residential Living Environments and Placement Stability Scale (ROLES) is an open-ended assessment of the type of living arrangements a child encountered during the assessment period and length of time in each, along with an assessment of the relative restrictiveness of each setting. The ROLES, as used in the outcome study, is an adaptation of the scale developed by Hawkins, Almeida, Fabry, and Reitz (1992).

Educational performance and juvenile justice contacts.   Academic performance over the past 90 days was rated on a 4-point scale ranging from 1 (*failing*; GPA 0%–59%), 2 (*below average*; GPA 60%–69%), 3 (*average;* GPA 70%–79%), to 4 (*above average;* 80%–100%). School attendance over the past 90 days was assessed on a 5-point scale ranging from 1 (*not attending;* 0%) to 5 (*attends regularly*; 76%–100%). Juvenile justice contacts were defined as the number of contacts a child had with law enforcement as a result of legal infractions.

Data Collection

Initial descriptive information on children and families receiving system-of-care services was collected through in-person interviews with caregivers, or by completion of questionnaires by case workers based on intake records. Diagnoses were based on criteria from the *DSM–IV* and were obtained from management information systems, case records, or clinician assessments.

Caregivers of children or adolescents eligible for participation in the outcome study were approached and consent was obtained. Baseline in-person interviews were conducted with caregivers and adolescents 11 years of age or older by either caseworkers or data collectors within 30 days of entry into services. The baseline CBCL and YSR were administered during the intake procedure or as part of the baseline interviews and assessed children's symptoms during the preceding 6 months. The baseline CAFAS was completed by trained raters to reflect children's functioning during the same period. In most cases, these ratings were determined by clinicians who obtained information from multiple informants such as the children, caregivers, schools, and official records; in some cases, ratings were based on information obtained by structured interviews with the caregivers. At follow-up, the CBCL and YSR were administered either in the clinical setting or as a part of the follow-up interviews; the CAFAS was again completed by trained raters familiar with the children. Information about the children's educational status was largely collected from caregivers, although some communities collected school attendance and achievement information from school records. Juvenile justice data were collected through a combination of information from caregivers, review of juvenile justice records, and reports by parole officers. Data were entered into data tables by community evaluation staff and forwarded to the national evaluation office where they were converted to SPSS (Statistical Package for the Social Sciences, 1999) and aggregated for analysis.

Although study enrollment and data collection procedures were established nationally, each community customized aspects of the evaluation to meet local criteria or needs. For example, variations in local procedures were influenced by informed consent requirements, administration of additional local measures, data collection strategies, and available resources. Interview incentives provided to caregivers and youth varied according to local resources and preferences.

Data Analysis

Descriptive analyses were conducted on data collected at intake to examine characteristics of children and families entering system-of-care services. Analyses of differences in outcomes at intake based on characteristics of children and families were conducted using chi-square and *t*-test statistics as appropriate. Analyses of changes in outcomes over time were conducted using analysis of variance. Analyses of changes among children enrolled in system-of-care services to 2 years include only those groups of children and families from the outcome study sample who had complete data at four evaluation points (intake, 6 months, 1 year, and 2 years) for a particular analysis. In addition to clinical assessments, children's abilities to function in the home and community were assessed by examining stability of the living arrangements and contacts with the juvenile justice system across time. Children's abilities to function in school were assessed by analyzing changes in school performance and attendance over time using analysis of variance. Due to missing data and varying data collection procedures, the number of children for whom data were available varied across analyses.

RESULTS

Presentation and History

Diagnosis.   Of the 34,811 children in the descriptive sample for whom a primary diagnosis was reported, 42.9% displayed a disruptive behavior disorder

(29.3% conduct-related disorders, 13.6% attention deficit hyperactivity disorder); 26% were diagnosed with depression or dysthymia, 8.0% with an anxiety disorder, and 6.4% with an adjustment disorder. The remaining primary diagnostic categories (assigned to 7.8% of the sample) included substance use, 1.9%; abuse or neglect, 0.3%; personality disorders, 0.4%; learning disabilities, 0.8%; developmental disorders or autism, 1.5%; psychosis, 1.9%; and other diagnoses such as eating, somatic, or speech disorders, phobia, enuresis, or encopresis, 1.2%. Primary diagnoses were deferred for 8.9% of children. For the 10,127 children with co-occurring disorders (29.1%), the most prevalent secondary diagnoses included conduct-related disorders (18.0%), substance use (17.0%), depression or dysthymia (11.0%), and attention deficit hyperactivity disorder (10.0%). Secondary diagnoses were deferred for 17% of these children.

Referral source. Children entered the system of care through a variety of avenues. Among the 10,699 children for whom data were available, mental health agencies provided the largest proportion of referrals (22.0%), closely followed by schools (20.5%). Another 14.5% of children were referred from social service agencies, and 13.7% were directed to the system of care through the courts and correctional institutions. Those referred by caregivers or themselves accounted for 16.0% of the children. There was a significant difference in the racial and ethnic distributions of the children referred by their parents or themselves (i.e., self-referral) and those referred by external sources such as schools or mental health agencies (i.e., external referral), $\chi^2(6, N = 10,402) = 241.74, p < .001$. In the self-referral group, 70.9% of the children were White; 16.1% were African American; 7.2% were Hispanic; 4.6% were American Indian or Alaskan Native; and 1.1% were Asian, Pacific Islander, or Native Hawaiian. In contrast, 54.5% of the children in the external referral group were White, whereas 14.8% were African American; 25.5% were Hispanic; 1.7% were American Indian or Alaskan Native; and 3.5% were Asian, Pacific Islander, or Native Hawaiian. Within race categories, Whites and African Americans reported self-referral in equal proportions (5.5% and 4.7%, respectively). Equal proportions of Hispanics and Asians, Pacific Islanders, and Native Hawaiians also reported self-referral (1.3% for both categories), but in lower proportions than Whites or African Americans. American Indians, and Alaskan Natives had the highest proportion reporting self-referral (10.9%).

Risk factors. Among 10,467 children, 67.2% were described by their caregivers as having experienced one or more child risk factors including physical abuse, sexual abuse, previous psychiatric hospitalization, sexual abusiveness, suicide attempt, drug and alcohol use, and a history of running away. Of children who experienced multiple child-risk factors prior to intake, 19.2% had experienced two such risk factors prior to intake whereas 21.0% had experienced three or more.

Family risk factors including family history of mental illness, psychiatric hospitalization, felony convictions, substance use, and family violence were reported for 82.6% of 10,655 children. Family histories of substance use, violence, and mental illness were the most frequently reported family risk factors. Multiple family risk factors were reported for most families at intake: 21.1% had two family risk factors, and 40.5% experienced at least three family risk factors.

Clinical Characteristics

Table 1 presents descriptive data for clinical measures of child behavioral and emotional symptoms and child social functioning at intake, as measured by the CBCL, the YSR, and the CAFAS. Children in the longitudinal sample exhibited more externalizing behavior problems than internalizing behavior problems based on both caregiver and youth reports. For the CBCL at intake, 52.0% of the children scored above the clinical range for internalizing behaviors, 65.6% attained scores in the clinical range for externalizing behaviors, and 69.4% of the children attained scores in the clinical range on the CBCL total problem scale. For the YSR, the percentages were considerably lower: 25.9% for internalizing behaviors, 39.4% for externalizing behaviors, and 35.7% for total problems. This discrepancy between CBCL and YSR scores has been reported frequently in the literature (Handwerk, Larzelere, Soper, & Friman, 1999; Stephens & Holden, 2001).

Child and family risk factors were associated with total problem scores on the CBCL at intake: child risk factors, $F(3, 6397) = 82.35$, $p < .001$; family risk factors, $F(3, 6510) = 44.91$, $p < .001$. For child risk factors, children with three or more risk factors had significantly higher total problems scores ($M = 71.3$, $SD = 10.4$) than those with two risk factors ($M = 68.9$, $SD = 10.7$), one risk factor ($M = 67.8$, $SD = 10.6$), and no risk factors ($M = 65.6$, $SD = 10.5$). All differences were significant at $p < .001$, except for the difference between one risk factor and two risk factors, which was significant at $p < .02$. For family risk factors, children with three or more risk factors had significantly higher total problems scores ($M = 69.2$, $SD = 10.6$) than those with two risk factors ($M = 68.5$, $SD = 10.2$), one risk factor ($M = 67.6$, $SD = 10.6$), and no risk factors ($M = 64.9$, $SD = 10.9$). All differences were significant at $p < .001$, except for the difference between one risk factor and two risk factors and the difference between two risk factors and three or more risk factors that were not significant. In addition, intake CBCL total problem scores differed by age groups, $F(2, 11205) = 54.59$, $p < .001$. Children 16 and older exhibited significantly fewer behavioral and emotional problems ($M = 65.2$, $SD = 11.9$) than those 12 to 15 years old ($M = 67.8$, $SD = 10.9$) and those 5 to 11 years old ($M =$

TABLE 1
Mean CBCL and YSR *T* Scores and Mean CAFAS Scores
at Intake for Children 5 Years and Older

Variable	n	M	SD
CBCL			
Total problems	11,208	67.5	11.1
Internalizing problems	11,200	63.3	11.9
Externalizing problems	11,211	67.1	11.8
YSR			
Total problems	7,027	58.8	11.8
Internalizing problems	7,017	55.8	12.2
Externalizing problems	7,021	60.2	11.7
CAFAS			
Total	14,525	92.3	45.9
Home	14,448	17.6	10.6
School or work	14,379	19.1	10.6
Community	14,419	9.7	11.3
Behavior toward others	14,519	16.1	8.9
Moods and emotions	14,491	14.0	9.4
Self-harmful behavior	14,341	6.7	10.0
Substance abuse behavior	14,477	5.4	10.0
Thinking	14,478	4.3	7.9

Note. CBCL = Child Behavior Checklist; YSR = Youth Self-Report; CAFAS = Child and Adolescent Functional Assessment Scale.

68.2, $SD = 10.8$). Similar results were observed for YSR *total problems* at intake with regard to the influence of risk factors and age.

As Table 1 shows, among children enrolled in the outcome study, the average total CAFAS score at intake was 92.3 ($SD = 45.9$), an average score near the top of the moderate range. Slightly more than 66% of children received school role scores in the moderate or severe range. On the home role subscale, 56.8% of children had moderate or severe scores, and 58.3% of children had scores in the moderate or severe categories on the behavior toward others subscale.

CAFAS scores differed according to a child's gender, age, history of risk factors, and diagnoses. Boys exhibited greater functional impairment than girls in CAFAS total scores (boys: $M = 94.8, SD = 45.2$; girls: $M = 87.5, SD = 46.8$), $t(10061) = 9.04, p < .001$. This was true in each of the three domains of role performance (i.e., home, school, community), particularly at school (boys: $M = 20.4, SD = 10.0$; girls: $M = 16.8, SD = 11.4$), $t(9170) = 18.98, p < .001$, and in the community (boys: $M = 10.9, SD = 11.6$; girls: $M = 7.4, SD = 10.3$), $t(11384) = 18.63, p < .001$. Likewise, older children were more functionally impaired in their CAFAS total scores than were younger children, $F(2, 14522) = 603.73, p < .001$. This was accounted for predominately by the community role performance scores that were considerably higher for older children; children over the age of 15 had a mean community role performance score of 14.96 (SD = 11.88) compared to a mean score of 11.64 (SD = 11.63) for 12- to 15-year-olds and a mean score of 4.92 (SD = 8.47) for those of children between the ages of 5 and 11 years old. This difference is, however, expected because CAFAS scores are to some extent affected by the age of the child. The community role scale assesses behaviors such as stealing, robbery, intentionally playing with fire, and damage to community property. Older children have greater access to the larger community in which these behaviors are enacted and are therefore more likely to engage in these behaviors than younger children.

Children's histories serve as important predictors of CAFAS scores at intake: for child risk factors, $F(3, 7629)$ = 454.23, $p < .001$; for family risk factors, $F(3, 7733)$ = 56.39, $p < .001$. Those children with no child risk factors at intake had significantly lower mean total CAFAS scores (M = 68.5, SD = 37.0) than those with one risk factor (M = 85.2, SD = 41.1), two risk factors (M = 97.4, SD = 43.3), and three or more risk factors (M = 115.7, SD = 45.4); the same trend was seen for the number of family risk factors. In addition, certain primary diagnoses predicted higher CAFAS scores at intake, $F(3, 10409)$ = 81.23, $p < .001$. For example, mean total CAFAS scores at intake for children with a primary diagnosis of depression (M = 100.1, SD = 46.5) or conduct-related disorder (M = 98.4, SD = 44.6) were significantly higher than for those children with a primary diagnosis of attention deficit hyperactivity disorder (M = 84.8, SD = 35.9) or anxiety (M = 84.8, SD = 43.8).

Clinical Outcomes

Change in behavioral and emotional symptoms.   Figure 1 depicts the significant decrease in CBCL scores from intake to 2 years for internalizing problems, $F(3, 2379)$ = 70.29, $p < .001$; externalizing problems, $F(3, 2376)$ = 73.73, $p < .001$; and total problems scores, $F(3, 2379)$ = 99.79, $p < .001$. The reliable change index (RCI; Jacobson, Roberts, Berns, & McGlinchey, 1999; Jacobson & Truax, 1991; Speer & Greenbaum, 1995) was also used to assess individual behavioral and emotional change over time. This statistic compares a child's scores at two different points in time and indicates whether a change in scores shows clinically significant improvement, stability, or deterioration. Figure 2 displays the RCI results from intake to 2 years for children's CBCL total problem scores. From intake to 2 years, 44.8% of children exhibited clinically significant improvement. Of those, 56.7% fell below the clinical cutoff for CBCL total problems T scores at 2 years compared to 6.7% at intake.

Change in functional assessment.   Children enrolled in the systems of care experienced moderate improvement in their CAFAS role performance score

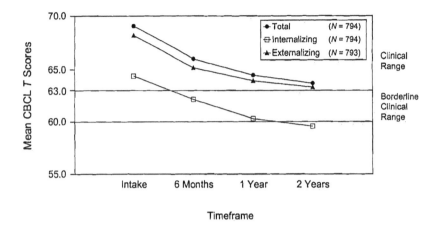

FIGURE 1   Mean Child Behavior Checklist total, internalizing and externalizing problems *T* scores at intake, 6 months, 1 year, and 2 years for children ages 5 and older.

from intake to 2 years. As seen in Figure 3, total CAFAS scores decreased substantially from intake to 2 years for children enrolled in systems of care, $F(3, 3324) = 58.99, p < .001$. The largest decline in total CAFAS scores occurred during the first 6 months after intake into services for both boys and girls. Although boys had somewhat higher total CAFAS scores than girls, both improved significantly from intake to 2 years. Because the CAFAS lacks psychometric data from a normative sample, the RCI cannot be calculated in the same manner as it is for the CBCL and YSR (Jacobson & Truax, 1991). Instead, a 20-point change in the CAFAS total score was defined as clinically significant. This translates into 0.44 standard deviations. Using this criterion, 49.5% of children exhibited clinically significant change from intake to 2 years.

Functional Outcomes

Stability of living arrangements.   Overall, the stability of living arrangements increased among children remaining in system-of-care services from intake to 2 years ($N = 10,642$). Among the 10,082 children who provided data at baseline, 57.5% reported only one living arrangement for the year prior to intake, with the remaining 42.5% reporting two or more living arrangements for that same period. Among the 4,019 children who provided data at the 12-month follow-up wave, the percentage who reported only one living arrangement in the six months prior to the interview increased to 72.9%, and among the 1,816 children with data at the

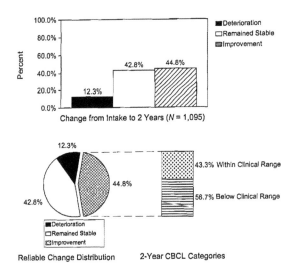

FIGURE 2   Percentage of children whose mean Child Behavior Checklist total problems *T* scores improved, remained stable, or deteriorated from intake to 2 years and percentage of children who improved within or below clinical range.

24-month follow-up wave, 73.6% reported only one living arrangement during the year prior to the interview.

Educational placement and performance.   Overall, school performance and attendance improved for both boys and girls from intake to 2 years after intake into services. The time main effect was significant for school attendance, $F(3, 2961) = 3.82, p < .01$, and school performance, $F(3, 1968) = 8.72, p < .001$. Improvements were continuous to 1 year, with less improvement in school performance and a decline in attendance from 1 year to 2 years.

Contacts with law enforcement.   Overall, contacts with law enforcement decreased among children in systems of care from intake to 2 years ($N = 8,008$). Among the 7,724 children who provided data at baseline, 29.5% reported one or more contacts with law enforcement as a result of one or more violations of the law during the year prior to entering system-of-care services. Among the 2,968 children with data at the 12-month follow-up wave, 20.2% reported one or more contacts with law enforcement in the 6 months prior to the interview, and among the 1,417 children with data at the 24-month follow-up wave, 20.7% reported one or more contacts with law enforcement in the prior year.

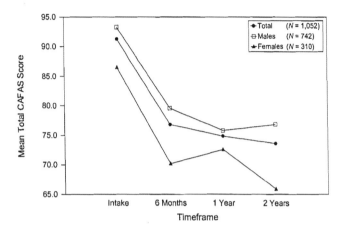

FIGURE 3   Mean total Child and Adolescent Functional Assessment Scale score for total
sample, boys, and girls at intake, 6 months, 1 year, and 2 years.

DISCUSSION

Children and youth who entered system-of-care services in communities receiving
grants in 1993 and 1994 were in some ways similar to children with serious emotional disturbances described in other studies (Bickman, Summerfelt, Firth, &
Douglas, 1997; Greenbaum et al., 1996; Kandel et al., 1997). Most of the children
were boys, and entry into services in early adolescence predominated. The majority
of children were diagnosed with disruptive behavior disorders or depression; entered services with considerable personal, familial, and social risk factors; and were
challenged by serious behavioral problems and impaired social functioning. For
the subgroup of children who remained in services over 2 years, considerable improvement in functioning and in emotional and behavioral symptoms was observed.

Children entered services through referrals from across the major child serving
sectors, in keeping with system-of-care program goals. Minority children entering
services were overrepresented when compared to population statistics (U.S. Census Bureau, 2000), reflecting the ethnic distribution of the funded communities.
When examining self and external referrals by ethnicity, findings were more complex than indicated by others (Takeuchi, Bui, & Kim,1993) who found that children and youth of color were more likely to be referred to services by external
agencies than White children. Although White children represented a larger percentage of those self referred, among those referred by external agencies, White
children and other children were referred in proportion to the ethnic distribution of
the sample. In addition, White families were no more likely to refer themselves

than African American families, and Native American families were most likely to initiate services themselves.

Children served by this program entered services with considerable challenges. These challenges included not only personal histories related to mental health, encounters with the juvenile justice system, unstable living situations, and difficulties in school. They also included difficult family circumstances that are impacted by high levels of poverty and the strains of single parenthood (McLoyd, 1991). When compared to other populations of children with mental health needs recently investigated (Bickman et al., 1995; Bickman et al., 1997), children served through this program showed greater functional impairment at intake, indicating a more severely challenged population. Nevertheless, these children made significant improvements in both behavior and functioning. These improvements included reduced contact with law enforcement, better grades and school attendance, and improved scores on clinical measures of behavioral and emotional problems and functional impairment.

As Farmer (2000) described, understanding which factors contribute to improvements in child and family outcomes is a complex matter. Because communities develop programs according to their own unique circumstances within the system-of-care framework, not all programs are exactly the same. As might be expected, not all communities had the same needs, served the same population, or had the same level of success at cross-agency collaboration. In addition, according to the principles guiding service provision within the system-of-care framework, determination of appropriate services was customized to the needs of a particular child and family. Consequently, the intervention or services that each child received was unique. This customization in and of itself can be considered the intervention. Other factors that may influence the understanding of outcomes include the unique clinical characteristics of children (Liao, Manteuffel, Paulic, & Sondheimer, 2001), changes in children's behaviors and functioning that may occur as a result of developing maturity, and factors external to treatment interventions such as social conditions or the environments (e.g., schools) in which children spend much of their time. These factors may have implications for policy and treatment design, as discussed by Holden, De Carolis, and Huff (2002).

The limitations of the evaluation of these communities include factors related to study design that became clearer as the study progressed. Although assumptions were initially made that children would remain in services until they improved, and consequently would not need to be followed further, it was found that children and families entered and exited services and that information was needed about outcomes beyond the successes achieved while in services. Knowledge of children's successes in services in this study is therefore more complete over the short term, and children who remain continuously in services and in the evaluation for 2 or even 3 years, may be a unique group. Variations in study implementation due to local decision making also impacted data completeness; consequently, it cannot be assumed that data were missing randomly or that the sample of children for whom data are available are representative of the communities served. In addition, this evaluation was not intended to be a randomized controlled trial, limiting our understanding of the impact of system change and service delivery on children's outcomes.

As a result of this experience, the evaluation design was changed when additional communities were funded. Changes in design include assessing children in and out of services, conducting comparison studies that examine system-of-care and non-system-of-care communities with greater attention to service delivery at the practice level, and examining the effectiveness of specific clinical treatments within the system-of-care framework. Understanding effectiveness of service provision is critical, yet the evaluation of community level effectiveness is a complex undertaking (Farmer, 2000; Holden, Friedman, & Santiago, 2001; Weisz, 2000). Success in this endeavor will require further integration of what are now relatively disparate literatures on the efficacy of clinical interventions and the effectiveness of community-based services.

ACKNOWLEDGMENTS

Work on this article was supported by Contract Numbers 280–97–8014, 280–99–8023, and 280– 00–8040 with the Child and Family Branch of the Center for Mental Health Services in the federal Substance Abuse and Mental Health Services Administration, United States Department of Health and Human Services.

REFERENCES

Achenbach, T. M. (1991a). *Manual for the Child Behavior Checklist 14–18 and 1991 Profile.* Burlington, VT: University Associates in Psychiatry.
Achenbach, T. M. (1991b). *Manual for the Youth Self-Report 11–18 and 1991 Profile.* Burlington, VT: University Associates in Psychiatry.
American Psychiatric Association. (1994). *Diagnostic and statistical manual of mental disorders* (4th ed.). Washington, DC: Author.
Bickman, L., Guthrie, P. R., Foster, E. M., Lambert, W., Summerfelt, W. T., Breda, C. S., & Heflinger, C. A. (1995). *Evaluating managed mental health services: The Fort Bragg experiment.* New York: Plenum.
Bickman, L., Summerfelt, W., Firth, J., & Douglas, S. (1997). The Stark County evaluation project: Baseline results of a randomized experiment. In C. Nixon & D. Northrup (Eds.), *Evaluating mental health services* (pp. 231–258). Thousand Oaks, CA: Sage.
Farmer, E. M. Z. (2000). Issues confronting effective services in systems of care. *Children and Youth Services Review, 22,* 627–650.
Greenbaum, P. E., Dedrick, R. F., Friedman, F. M., Kutash, K., Brown, E. D., Lardieri, S. P., & Pugh, A. M. (1996). National adolescent and child treatment study (NACTS): Outcomes for children with serious emotional and behavioral disturbance. *Journal of Emotional and Behavioral Disorders, 4,* 130–146.

Handwerk, M. L., Larzelere, R. E., Soper, S. H., & Friman, P. C. (1999). Parent and child discrepancies in reporting severity of problem behaviors in three out-of-home settings. *Psychological Assessment, 11*, 14–23.

Hawkins, R. P., Almeida, M. C., Fabry, B., & Reitz, A. L. (1992). A scale to measure restrictiveness of living environments for troubled children and youths. *Hospital and Community Psychiatry, 43*, 54–58.

Hodges, K. (1990). *The Child and Adolescent Functional Assessment Scale (CAFAS)*. Unpublished manuscript.

Holden, E. W., De Carolis, G., & Huff, B. (2002/this issue). Policy implications of the National Evaluation of the Comprehensive Community Mental Health Services for Children and Their Families program. *Children's Services: Social Policy, Research, and Practice, 5*, 57–65.

Holden, E. W., Friedman, R. M., & Santiago, R. L. (2001). Overview of the national evaluation of the Comprehensive Community Mental Health Services for Children and Their Families program. *Journal of Emotional and Behavioral Disorders, 9*, 4–12.

Jacobson, N. S., Roberts, L. J., Berns, S. B., & McGlinchey, J. B. (1999). Methods for defining and determining the clinical significance of treatment effects: Description, application and alternatives. *Journal of Consulting and Clinical Psychology, 67*, 300–307.

Jacobson, N. S., & Truax, P. (1991). Clinical significance: A statistical approach to defining meaningful change in psychotherapy research. *Journal of Consulting and Clinical Psychology, 59*, 12–19.

Kandel, D. B., Johnson, J. G., Bird, H. R., Canino, G., Goodman, S. H., Lahey, B. B., Regier, D. A., & Schwab-Stone, M. (1997). Psychiatric disorders associated with substance use among children and adolescents: Findings from the methods for the epidemiology of child and adolescent mental disorders (MECA) study. *Journal of Abnormal Child Psychology, 25*, 121–132.

Liao, Q., Manteuffel, B., Paulic, C., & Sondheimer, D. (2001). Describing the population of adolescents served in systems of care. *Journal of Emotional and Behavioral Disorders, 9*, 13–29.

McLoyd, V. C. (1991). The strain of living poor. In A. C. Huston (Ed.), *Children in poverty* (pp. 105–135). New York: Cambridge University Press.

Speer, D. C., & Greenbaum, P. E. (1995). Five methods for computing significant individual client change and improvement rates: Support for an individual growth curve approach. *Journal of Consulting and Clinical Psychology, 63*, 1044–1048.

Statistical Package for the Social Sciences (SPSS Version 9.0) [Computer software]. (1999). Chicago: SPSS, Inc.

Stephens, R. L., & Holden, E. W. (2001). Accounting for differences in youth and caregiver reports of behavioral and emotional symptoms. In C. Newman, C. Liberton, K. Kutash, & R. M. Friedman (Eds.), *The 13th Annual Research Conference Proceedings: A System of Care for Children's Mental Health: Expanding the Research Base* (pp. 329–332). Tampa: University of South Florida, The Louis de la Parte Florida Mental Health Institute, Research and Training Center for Children's Mental Health.

Stroul, B. A., & Friedman, R. M. (1986). *A system of care for children and youth with severe emotional disturbances* (Rev. ed.). Washington, DC: Georgetown University Child Development Center, CASSP Technical Assistance Center.

Takeuchi, D. T., Bui, K. V., & Kim, L. (1993). The referral of minority adolescents to community mental health centers. *Journal of Health and Social Behavior, 34*, 153–164.

U.S. Census Bureau. (2000). *Resident population estimates of the United States by sex, race, and Hispanic origin: April 1, 1990 to July 1, 1999, with short-term projection to July 1, 2000* [On-line]. Retrieved August 25, 2000 from the World Wide Web: http://www.census.gov/population/estimates/nation/intfile3-1.txt

U.S. Department of Health and Human Services. (1999). *Mental Health: A Report of the Surgeon General*. Rockville, MD: U.S. Department of Health and Human Services, Substance Abuse and Mental

Health Services Administration, Center for Mental Health Services, National Institutes of Health, National Institute of Mental Health.

Weisz, J. R. (2000). Lab–clinic differences and what we can do about them: I. The clinic-based treatment development model. *Clinical Child Psychology Newsletter, 15*(1), 1–3, 10.

CHILDREN'S SERVICES: SOCIAL POLICY, RESEARCH, AND PRACTICE, 5(1), 21–36

The Impact of Managed Care on Systems of Care That Serve Children With Serious Emotional Disturbances and Their Families

Beth A. Stroul

Management & Training Innovations
McLean, VA

Sheila A. Pires

Human Service Collaborative
Washington, DC

Mary I. Armstrong

Department of Child & Family Studies
Louis de la Parte Florida Mental Health Institute
University of South Florida

Susan Zaro

ORC Macro
Atlanta, GA

A qualitative case study approach was used to evaluate the impact of managed care reforms on a select sample of systems of care funded by the Comprehensive Community Mental Health Services for Children and Their Families Program. Analyses indicated that the system-of-care philosophy and approach could be maintained in a managed care environment under the right circumstances. These circumstances include (a) the preexistence of a system-of-care philosophy prior to the integration of managed care, (b) stakeholder involvement in managed care planning and implementation, (c) use of a broad array of providers and sufficient support for case manage-

Requests for reprints should be sent to Susan Zaro, ORC Macro, 3 Corporate Square, Suite 370, Atlanta, GA 30329. E-mail: zaro@macroint.com

ment and care coordination activities, (d) identification and support of high utilizer groups within the managed care system, and (e) financial compatibility between managed care and systems of care.

During the past decade, there has been progress throughout the country in the implementation and financing of community-based systems of care for children and adolescents with serious emotional disturbances and their families. This has taken place primarily in the public sector, for children with the most serious needs (Cole, 1996; Cole & Poe, 1993; Davis, Yelton, & Katz-Leavy, 1993; Lourie, Katz-Leavy, De Carolis, & Quinlan, 1996; Stroul, 1996a). The system-of-care philosophy emphasizes a broad array of services, including (a) a comprehensive range of intensive nonresidential and residential services and supports; (b) treatment in the least restrictive, most appropriate setting; (c) individualized and flexible treatment and services; (d) interagency collaboration among the various agencies and systems that share responsibility for children and youth with serious emotional disorders; (e) family involvement in planning and delivery of services; and (f) culturally competent services (Stroul & Friedman, 1986). State Medicaid programs increasingly have been used to fund services in systems of care (Behar, 1996; Meyers, 1994). In addition, a major source of funding for these systems has come through the Comprehensive Community Mental Health Services for Children and Their Families Program (CMHS), a federal program established by the Center for Mental Health Services.

These system-building activities are not occurring in a vacuum. Rather, they are taking place in a larger environment that is undergoing swift and dramatic change. One such change is the rapid and widespread implementation of managed care in health and human services, in particular the application of managed care technologies to behavioral health service delivery (Pires, Armstrong, & Stroul, 1999; Pires, Stroul, & Armstrong, 2000; Pires et al., 1996). Soaring health care costs in the 1980s led to a number of cost containment strategies, most of which were subsumed under the general heading of managed care (Kent & Hersen, 2000). First seen primarily in private sector commercial insurance plans, rising health care costs also have resulted in the movement of state Medicaid programs away from fee-for-service plans and toward managed care (U.S. General Accounting Office, 1995). These changes have affected behavioral health services as well as physical health care. In a recently conducted survey of state-managed care initiatives affecting behavioral health services, 42 states (including the District of Columbia) reported involvement in publicly financed managed care activity affecting behavioral health services for children, adolescents, and their families (Stroul, Pires, & Armstrong, in press).

With the advent of managed care, system-of-care proponents have raised questions as to the implications for service delivery. Of concern is (a) whether progress in building systems of care is in jeopardy, (b) whether the system-of-care philosophy will be abandoned, (c) whether use of Medicaid to support system-of-care components and wraparound services will be curtailed, and (d) whether access to appropriate and high quality behavioral health services (mental health and substance abuse) for children and adolescents with serious disorders and their families will be compromised (Stroul, 1996b). Other questions that have been raised include (a) whether the advent of managed care could result in a regression to a traditional insurance model of covering a limited number of services for a limited amount of time, (b) whether children with serious disorders will be underserved due to insufficient incentives in managed care systems to serve the so-called "high utilizers" of services, (c) whether provider networks including nontraditional programs and providers will become less viable, and (d) whether the needs of culturally diverse children and families will receive less attention under new managed care systems (Stroul, Pires, & Armstrong, 1998a).

Despite their apprehensions about managed care, system-of-care proponents also have recognized opportunities to improve service delivery and to advance system-of-care goals presented by managed care reforms. Managed care reforms may offer opportunities to redesign the service system to expand the array of services covered by Medicaid, adding a range of intermediate services and supports and increased accountability with a greater focus on outcome and quality measurement (Stroul et al., 1998a). Managed care reforms also could mean ending arbitrary benefit limits as a strategy to manage costs, promoting the routine use of empirically based service approaches, improving efficiencies through capitated financing, and improving coordination of health and mental health care (Ridgely, Giard, & Shern, 1999).

This study was designed to explore (a) the "intersection" of managed care and systems of care in the CMHS-funded sites and to assess the impact of managed care initiatives on the development and operation of local systems of care in selected CMHS-funded sites; (b) the impact of managed care initiatives on children and adolescents with emotional disorders and their families through the lens of various stakeholders in the sites; (c) how different groups of stakeholders view managed care reforms, the positive effects and the problems that have been created; and (d) which aspects of the structure, design, organization, and characteristics of managed care systems have facilitated or created problems for mental health service delivery to children, adolescents, and their families.

METHOD

Given the exploratory nature of this work, a qualitative case study design with multiple cases was employed. This method allows for the empirical investigation of contemporary phenomena within a real-life context using multiple sources of evidence (Yin, 1984).

Review of Information

The study began with a review of information related to managed care collected by the CMHS program's national evaluator, Macro International Inc., during their visits in 1996 to 27 CMHS-funded sites. The information included notes and site visit reports taken from the managed care section of the system assessment component of the national evaluation that addressed the current status of managed care planning or implementation and the effects or anticipated effects of managed care on the system of care. In addition, data and findings were reviewed from the Health Care Reform Tracking Project, a national study initiated in 1995 to track and analyze the impact of public sector managed care reforms on children and adolescents with emotional and substance abuse disorders and their families. This included the results of the 1995 State Survey and preliminary observations emanating from the 1997 Impact Analysis (Pires et al., 1996; Stroul, Pires, & Armstrong, 1998b; Stroul et al., 1997).

Selection of a Sample of Sites

At the time of these reviews, 3 of the 27 CMHS-funded sites had no plans for managed care on the horizon, 12 sites were in the planning phase for managed care, 7 sites had only recently implemented managed care, and 5 sites had some degree of experience with managed care reforms in their site. From the group of 12 sites with sufficient experience with managed care such that effects could be discerned, 5 sites were selected for inclusion in the study with the goal of achieving a sample with some diversity in stage of implementation of managed care, characteristics of managed care reforms, approach to system-of-care development, and geographic location. Two sites were selected for telephone interviews—Lane County, Oregon, and the state of Rhode Island—and three sites were selected for site visits—Milwaukee, Wisconsin; Solano County, California; and San Mateo County, California. At the time of the telephone interviews and site visits, Lane County had recently implemented managed care whereas the other four sites included in the sample had implemented managed care for a minimum of 1 year and had a substantial base of experience.

Data Collection

Data were collected using telephone and on-site interviews with multiple key stakeholders in each of the five sites. Using the experience of the Health Care Reform Tracking Project, interview guides were developed to provide a basic structure and to enhance consistency in the information gathered across sites. The guides addressed a number of areas of inquiry, including a general assessment of managed care reforms; the impact of design and structural characteristics of managed care systems; and the impact on service delivery, systems of care, and providers. Managed care impacts on family involvement, cultural competence, interagency relations, financing, and accountability of managed care systems were also addressed.

The multidisciplinary interviewing team that conducted both telephone and on-site interviews was knowledgeable about systems of care for children with emotional disorders and about behavioral health managed care, with experience in the research, policy, and practice arenas. A team of two interviewers conducted the interviews when possible to avoid the introduction of a particular discipline's bias. Team debriefings also reduced the possibility of such a bias while enhancing the richness of the data. The teams followed written procedures for collecting relevant documentation both prior to and during the interviews.

A series of telephone interviews was conducted with key informants from Lane County and Rhode Island in 1997. Interviewees typically included the site director and one or two additional individuals from the site. Site visits to Milwaukee, Solano County, and San Mateo County also were conducted in 1997. During a two-day site visit, interviews were conducted with a wide variety of stakeholder groups, including site director and key project staff; families; representatives of the behavioral health managed care organization (MCO); children's mental health service providers; care managers and clinicians; and representatives of the child welfare, juvenile justice, and education systems. Where possible, interviews were conducted in group settings to obtain a balanced set of observations and perspectives, both within and across stakeholder groups. Approximately seven to eight group interviews were conducted in each site, ranging from 2 to 3 hr each; the total number of individuals interviewed per site ranged from 25 to 40.

Data Analysis

Following the telephone interviews and site visits, a case study report was prepared for each site. The individual case studies summarized findings within each of the dimensions included in the site visit protocol, detailing positive and negative effects of managed care reforms based on the perceptions and assessments of multiple stakeholders. These reports were sent to the site directors for each site for review of factual accuracy and then revised to incorporate feedback from the site directors.

Following completion of the case study reports, data were then analyzed across sites to synthesize findings, identify trends, and raise critical issues. In addition to a qualitative analysis of the information included in the individual case study reports, a systematic process was used to compare findings across sites. Within each dimension, key issues were identified and the findings related to each of these issues were "tallied" across sites. For example, in exploring the impact of managed care reforms on service delivery, the five sites were rated in numerous areas, including such issues as whether the managed care reform resulted in significant expansion of the array of services available in the community; whether the managed care reform facilitated or impeded the provision of home and community-based services and individualized, flexible care; and whether access to appropriate services in the least restrictive environment was improved. Similarly in the dimension exploring the impact of managed care reforms on family involvement, each site was rated on issues such as whether the managed care reforms have supported family involvement in treatment planning and service delivery for their own children and whether family members of children with behavioral health disorders were involved in managed care planning, advisory, and oversight structures at the system management level.

Although the sample of sites was small, the ratings yielded a summary of the effects of managed care reforms across the five CMHS-funded sites in key issue areas related to the effects of managed care reforms on children and adolescents with emotional disorders and their families and on the systems of care that serve them. In addition to these summary ratings, the qualitative material included in the case studies was a rich source of descriptive, explanatory, and interpretive information. A comprehensive report was developed blending the information derived from this data analysis process (Stroul et al., 1998a).[1]

RESULTS

Due to the small sample of sites and the distinct differences among them, the analysis describes, compares, and explains the experience of these sites without drawing inappropriate cross-site conclusions.

Systems of Care and Managed Care: Compatibility Issues

Integration of managed care and systems of care.   The degree of integration of managed care systems and systems of care varied considerably across sites. The degree of integration ranged from the system of care being fully incorporated in the managed care system as an expanded benefit for children with serious disorders in Lane County, to being a specialized carve-out for children with serious

---

[1]For a copy of this report, contact ORC Macro, Attn: Leza Young, 3 Corporate Square, Suite 370, Atlanta, GA 30329, (404) 321-3211, e-mail: Lyoung@macroint.com

disorders in Milwaukee, to being considered a tier or a level in the overall system for children with serious disorders in San Mateo County. In two sites, Rhode Island and Solano County, the systems of care were not integrated with managed care and essentially functioned separately. The lack of integration was regarded by stakeholders as problematic in both sites, causing duplication, difficulty tracking children across the entire continuum of care, confusion for families, and discontinuities across parallel operating systems.

Goals.   Cost-related goals for managed care systems (e.g., containing costs, reducing costs, or improving the cost-effectiveness of service delivery) were mentioned by respondents in all five sites but were not necessarily presented as the overriding goals for the managed care reforms. In all five sites, stakeholders reported that improving access to services was a significant goal as well. Other goals included (a) ensuring access specifically to mental health services for Medicaid recipients, many of whom were not receiving care previously; (b) strengthening primary care for pregnant women and children; (c) normalizing medical care for the Medicaid population; (d) decreasing emergency room use; (e) expanding access to preventive health care services; and (f) improving health outcomes for children.

Aside from improving access, the goals of the managed care reforms in the sites where the existing systems of care were not integrated with the managed care systems were not considered by respondents to be consistent with system-of-care goals. Stakeholders in Rhode Island perceived that the managed care system focused on short-term services and did not include the longer term, more intensive services and supports needed by children and adolescents with more serious disorders that are the essence of systems of care. Stakeholders in Solano County considered the system of care to be a different, more intensive level of care that was beyond the managed care system. In contrast, in the other three CMHS sites where integration between the two systems existed, the goals of the managed care reforms were considered by stakeholders to be consistent with system-of-care goals.

Services to children with serious disorders.   The varying integration across the systems of care and managed care systems led to varying arrangements for service delivery for children with serious disorders and varying issues raised by interviewees. Few issues were raised in Milwaukee where the managed care system and system of care were one and the same. Nor has managed care reform had a significant impact in San Mateo County where the high utilizer group (those with serious disorders) were served through the system-of-care tier, with services provided by county employees on a fee-for-service basis. In Lane County, services to children with serious disorders were provided by the system of care that was embedded in the managed care system as an expanded benefit for this group. Respondents noted that the managed care reform has actually impeded services to this population and threatened the future of the system of care due to the severe fiscal cuts accompanying the reform. The managed care system in Rhode Island generally did not provide a full array of services appropriate for children with serious emotional disorders because resources were not sufficient. Sizable behavioral health resources remained outside of the managed care system, and only a small portion of the capitation typically was allocated to behavioral health services by the MCOs.

MCOs.   In four of the five CMHS sites studied, the county mental health agency served as the MCO for the managed care system.[2] Respondents in these sites expressed greater confidence that public entities would be less likely to move to a strict, bottom-line, business orientation in implementing managed care, and would be less likely to abandon the system-of-care philosophy and previous progress in system development. In addition, public entities were perceived as invested in and accountable to the community, familiar with the Medicaid population, more likely to have extensive knowledge of the range and quality of service providers in the community, and more likely to have experience involving consumers and families at the system and service delivery levels. Finally, public entities were perceived as being under pressure to reinvest "savings" into expanding the array of services available. Clearly, stakeholders felt that the use of public agencies as MCOs was more compatible with systems of care. In contrast, the use of for-profit MCOs in Rhode Island was regarded by some stakeholders as problematic because these commercial MCOs were not sufficiently familiar with the Medicaid population, did not have experience serving children with serious emotional disturbances, had difficulty maintaining continuity of care, and were less likely to understand how to link treatment and community supports.

Clinical decision making and management mechanisms.   Stakeholders in one site, Rhode Island, complained about prior authorization management mechanisms used by the MCOs to control service utilization, describing them as cumbersome, time consuming, confusing, and creating barriers to access. In contrast, respondents in San Mateo County and Milwaukee reported that complaints about prior authorization and other management mechanisms were infrequent, and these mechanisms were not seen as conflicting with the mission or operation of the systems of care. In San Mateo County, the primary gatekeeping mechanism was the central in-

---

[2]In Solano County, approximately 10% of the population was assigned to Kaiser, a commercial managed care organization, to manage both physical and behavioral health care. The county mental health agency served as the managed care organization for behavioral health services for the vast majority of the population.

take process through a system-of-care team that was responsible for an initial assessment of needs and referral to the appropriate provider and level of care. None of the sites studied reported having level of care criteria to guide clinical decision making for children and adolescents with serious emotional disorders.

Capitation and case rates.   The level of funding available within a managed care system was a significant determinant of the ability of the system to provide the range and level of services needed by children and adolescents with emotional disorders, particularly those with more serious and complex problems. Thus, the resources allocated to behavioral health services for children are a factor in the "compatibility" of managed care with systems of care. Several concerns were raised by providers about rates across all five sites. Most notably, providers commented on reimbursement rates and case rates that were considered to be too low, particularly when coupled with the burdensome administrative and paperwork requirements associated with managed care.

In Milwaukee, Solano County, and Lane County, the MCOs were at full financial risk; risk pools involving funds set aside to cover unforeseen expenditures were in place in Solano and Lane Counties to help to manage risk. In Rhode Island, a risk sharing arrangement was implemented whereby after 30 outpatient visits, the state picked up 90% of the cost of care. In Lane County, a risk adjustment mechanism in the form of a higher capitation rate was adopted for children determined to need the highest level of care (i.e., the system of care). The higher rate reportedly was made possible by the blending of federal CMHS resources from the system-of-care program with the resources from the managed care system. However, the ability of the system to maintain this differential rate when federal grant funding ended was seriously questioned by stakeholders.

Policy making, planning, and system design.   One would assume that, at both the state and local levels, the greater the involvement of individuals with expertise in children's behavioral health services, the greater the likelihood that managed care reforms will be consistent with the system-of-care philosophy and approach. Examples of this are found in several of the CMHS sites. In Milwaukee, a 3-year planning process engaged key stakeholders and tested the approach. An extensive participatory process also was used in San Mateo County to design the managed care system. In Lane County, respondents reported that many individuals with expertise in children's mental health services participated in the planning process for the managed care system. In all three of these sites, system-of-care principles and approaches were integrated into the managed care systems.

Impact on System-of-Care Principles and Operations

Comprehensive array of services.   System-of-care development efforts, supported by CMHS grant funds in combination with other resources, have resulted in a significant expansion of the array of services available in these sites. The effect of managed care reforms on the service array varied. In Milwaukee, San Mateo County, and Solano County, respondents reported that managed care reforms further facilitated the provision of a broad array of mental health services, or at least did not negatively affect the range of services. This was attributed, in part, to the ability to control inpatient costs and to reinvest savings in the creation of additional community-based services. However, in Lane County, the fiscal cuts associated with the managed care reform reportedly resulted in a substantial reduction in both the range and capacity of children's mental health services from what existed previously. Stakeholders in Rhode Island felt that the managed care reform impeded the ability to provide a range of services because the benefit included in the managed care system was perceived as limited, providing primarily inpatient and office-based outpatient services.

Home- and community-based services and individualized, flexible care.   Consistent with observations about the range of services, stakeholders in both Lane County and Rhode Island suggested that managed care reforms and related fiscal cuts and the tendency to rely on more traditional services impeded the ability to provide home- and community-based services and individualized, flexible care—all critical to systems of care. In the Solano and San Mateo sites, respondents noted that managed care reforms had little effect on the provision of home and community-based services or individualized, flexible care because most home and community-based services were provided through the system of care. In Milwaukee, home- and community-based services and individualized care were the hallmarks of the managed system of care, which, unlike the other sites, was designed to exclusively serve a population of youngsters with serious disorders.

Access to the least restrictive, appropriate services.   Access to appropriate services and maximizing use of services in the least restrictive setting are key features of systems of care. In four of the five CMHS sites, general access to a basic level of behavioral health services was reported to have improved as a result of managed care reforms. Lane County is the only site in which stakeholders suggested that access to services was compromised by the managed care reform as a result of budget cuts, service reductions, and the exclusion of certain diagnoses (such as conduct disorders). Given the CMHS funding stream, one would not expect to find concerns about access to longer term, extended care services. However, concerns were found in Rhode Island and Lane County due to limited benefits and budget cuts, respectively.

Service coordination.   In three of the five sites, respondents observed that managed care reforms resulted in improvements in coordinating services for children and adolescents and their families. In both Solano and San Mateo Counties, the addition of a toll-free telephone number to serve as a central entry point to services was characterized as a vehicle for improving service coordination. In Solano County, the toll-free number and the care managers associated with this mechanism reportedly allowed for better tracking of children. Stakeholders in Milwaukee reported a strong, positive impact on service coordination for the most-in-need population, particularly with respect to coordination among mental health, child welfare, and juvenile justice services. In contrast, stakeholders in Rhode Island reported that the managed care reform made it more difficult to coordinate multiple services to children because the managed care system added more players to the mix, tended to focus on one service at a time rather than on multiple services, and operated independently from the system of care.

Milwaukee was the only site in which the managed care reform was credited with improvements in case management. As a managed system of care for children with serious disorders, case management was viewed as the lynchpin of Wraparound Milwaukee. Care coordination was considered a key function of Milwaukee's case managers, and caseloads were limited to eight. Stakeholders pointed out that much attention was devoted to the training and supervision of case managers as well as to retention issues such as salary levels, merit raises, and educational opportunities.

Interagency collaboration at the system management level.   Respondents in two of the sites stated that managed care reforms have resulted in improved collaboration among child-serving agencies at the system level. In Milwaukee, stakeholders indicated that a thoughtful and deliberate process involving the mental health, child welfare, and juvenile justice systems was used to design and implement the managed system of care and that this strengthened cross-system relations. Similarly, the implementation of managed care in San Mateo County was described as a vehicle for improving on the existing strong base of interagency collaboration and trust that had resulted from previous system-of-care development efforts. Interagency collaboration reportedly was not strengthened by managed care reforms in the other three sites, and respondents in two sites noted that problems related to interagency relations existed prior to managed care reforms and have persisted. In Lane County, respondents explained that the managed care reform resulted in increased tension across child-serving agencies due to fiscal cuts, service reductions, and greater controls on service delivery.

Family involvement.   Managed care reforms reportedly have not supported family involvement in service planning and delivery for their own children to the extent that the system-of-care philosophy prescribes. In Lane County, for example, stakeholders reported that the stress of implementing managed care and other factors have resulted in less emphasis on family involvement in service planning. In Rhode Island, respondents noted that family involvement was not mandated in contracts with MCOs, nor was there training for MCOs or providers on family involvement principles. Respondents in San Mateo County explained that family involvement in service planning and delivery was occurring within the system-of-care level but that managed care reform has had little impact on family involvement in other levels of care. An exception is Milwaukee, where according to all stakeholders, families (and youth when possible) were actively involved in the service planning process.

Cultural competence.   No significant effects on the overall level of cultural competence were associated with managed care reforms. Respondents in all of the CMHS sites observed that enhancing the cultural competence of services was a challenge that pre-existed managed care and remained a significant challenge for service delivery systems. Respondents in San Mateo County felt that the managed care reform had a positive impact because requirements for cultural competence were articulated within the managed care system; that is, the managed care system included requirements that providers be multilingual and represent a cultural mix appropriate to the cultural mix of the Medicaid population. Despite such requirements, however, recruitment of multilingual and culturally diverse providers remained difficult. Requirements for training in cultural competence were included in contracts in both San Mateo and Solano Counties. Similar requirements were included in Lane County's provider contracts as well as a mandate to offer special services needed by culturally diverse groups, such as translation and interpretation. In Milwaukee, respondents emphasized that improving cultural competence was an important goal, and a cultural diversity work group met on a regular basis. Special emphasis was placed on creating a culturally diverse provider network—40% of Milwaukee's care coordinators were reported to be from minority groups. Stakeholders in several of the sites reported that training in cultural competence was offered to MCOs and providers.

DISCUSSION

The adoption of managed care technologies to finance and deliver behavioral health services is continuing to spread rapidly. Additional states and counties are in the process of planning and implementing managed care reforms, and those with existing managed care systems are in the ongoing process of problem solving and incorporating refinements. Although the sample of sites in this study was small, the study has yielded important insights about the effects of managed care reforms and their compatibility with the goals and approaches espoused by the system-of-care philosophy. Further, the study has been a first step toward elucidating the effects of managed care reforms on evolving systems of care, based on stakeholder observations in a sample of CMHS-funded systems of care. In answer to the concerns raised by proponents about the risks of managed care reform, such as whether building systems of care is in jeopardy, whether the system-of-care philosophy will be abandoned, and whether access will be curtailed, this study has shown that a number of variables appear to influence how well managed care works with systems of care.

In the CMHS-funded sites, some managed care reforms have been initiated and designed primarily at the state level (Lane County and Rhode Island); others have been designed primarily at the local level (Milwaukee, San Mateo County, and Solano County). Whether planning occurs primarily at the state or local level, the involvement of stakeholders with expertise in children's behavioral health services and systems of care appeared to be a key factor.

Overall, systems of care and managed care systems were more likely to be compatible when an ongoing system development initiative and commitment to the system-of-care philosophy pre-existed managed care at the state or local levels and when stakeholders with expertise in systems of care for children's behavioral health care were closely involved in managed care planning and implementation. When these two preconditions were met, the managed care system was more likely to incorporate the system-of-care philosophy and approach in its benefit design and in its requirements and guidelines for MCOs and providers. Specifically, the system-of-care features that can be incorporated into managed care system design and requirements include the following: a broad array of home and community-based treatment options and support services, access to appropriate services in the least restrictive setting, individualized and flexible care, service coordination, interagency service planning, family involvement, and cultural competence.

The following factors also were important: (a) whether a broad array of providers was included in the managed care provider network; (b) whether provisions were incorporated into the managed care system to encourage, and to allow billing for, service coordination and interagency service planning activities; (c) whether clinical decision-making criteria and utilization management processes allowed for the provision of appropriate types and levels of care and did not excessively restrict flexibility in service delivery; and (d) whether incentives were structured to maximize access to treatment in the least restrictive, appropriate setting. Further, the system-of-care approach was more likely to prevail when MCOs—whether public or private—were familiar with the system-of-care philosophy and approach and knowledgeable about the needs of children and adolescents with emotional disorders and their families.

A critical issue was the way in which services for children with serious and complex needs (i.e., the high utilizer population) were handled within the managed care system. For example, the compatibility of systems of care and managed care was enhanced when managed care systems were responsible for extended care and include longer term, extended care services or when systems of care were incorporated into managed care systems as a level of care for children with serious disorders. If extended care services were not included in the managed care system, compatibility was enhanced if there were clear criteria for movement of children from managed care systems to systems of care and for coordination between the two.

Finally, the compatibility of systems of care and managed care was affected by the following issues: whether financial resources within the system were sufficient to provide the range and level of services needed by children and adolescents with emotional disorders and to prevent underservice, particularly of those children with serious disorders, and whether risk adjustment mechanisms were incorporated into managed care systems to prevent incentives for under serving children and adolescents with more serious and complex disorders.

There were examples, within this sample of CMHS-funded sites, which showed that the system-of-care philosophy and approaches (or aspects of it) can, in fact, be maintained in a managed care environment and, under the right circumstances, can be used to shape managed care systems. There were, however, also clear indications that without specific attention to and planning for children and adolescents with emotional disorders, many features of systems of care can be threatened with managed care reforms. Despite these threats, there was evidence in this sample of CMHS-funded sites of efforts to stay true to the system-of-care philosophy even in the context of major system changes such as managed care reforms.

ACKNOWLEDGMENTS

This research was funded by a contract to Macro International Inc. from the federal Center for Mental Health Services in the Substance Abuse and Mental Health Services Administration (280–94–0012).

The study would not have been possible without the cooperation and contributions of many individuals. We thank the many stakeholders who shared their perceptions, observations, and assessments with us during site visits and telephone interviews. Family members, providers, program managers, local behavioral health planners and administrators, MCOs, advocates, and others comprised the primary data source for this work. Their time and insights are appreciated. The directors of the local systems of care in each of the sites included in the study sample spent many additional hours planning and preparing for our work, and we acknowledge their invaluable assistance.

REFERENCES

Behar, L. (1996). Financing systems of care. In B. A. Stroul (Ed.), *Children's mental health: Creating systems of care in a changing society* (pp. 299–312). Baltimore: Brookes.

Cole, R. (1996). The Robert Wood Johnson Foundation's Mental Health Services Program for Youth. In B. A. Stroul (Ed.), *Children's mental health: Creating systems of care in a changing society* (pp. 235–248). Baltimore: Brookes.

Cole, R., & Poe, S. (1993). *Partnerships for care: Systems of care for children with serious emotional disturbances and their families.* Washington, DC: Washington Business Group on Health.

Davis, M., Yelton, S., & Katz-Leavy, J. (1993, March). *Unclaimed children revisited: The status of state children's mental health services.* Paper presented to the Sixth Annual Research Conference: A System of Care for Children's Mental Health: Expanding the Research Base, Tampa, FL.

Kent, A. J., & Hersen, M. (2000). An overview of managed mental health care: Past, present, and future. In. A. J. Kent & M. Hersen (Eds.), *A psychologist's proactive guide to managed mental health care* (pp. 3–19). Mahwah, NJ: Lawrence Erlbaum Associates, Inc.

Lourie, I., Katz-Leavy, J., De Carolis, G., & Quinlan, W. (1996). The role of the federal government. In B. A. Stroul (Ed.), *Children's mental health: Creating systems of care in a changing society* (pp. 99–114). Baltimore: Brookes.

Meyers, J. (1994). Financing strategies to support innovations in service delivery to children. *Journal of Clinical Child Psychology, 23,* 48–54.

Pires, S. A., Armstrong, M. I., & Stroul, B. A. (1999). *Health care reform tracking project: Tracking state health care reforms as they affect children and adolescents with behavioral health disorders and their families—1997–98 State Survey.* Tampa: University of South Florida, Louis de la Parte Florida Mental Health Institute, Department of Child and Family Studies, Research and Training Center for Children's Mental Health.

Pires, S. A., Stroul, B. A., & Armstrong, M. I. (2000). *Health care reform tracking project: Tracking state health care reforms as they affect children and adolescents with behavioral health disorders and their families—1999 Impact Analysis.* Tampa: University of South Florida, Louis de la Parte Florida Mental Health Institute, Department of Child and Family Studies, Research and Training Center for Children's Mental Health.

Pires, S., Stroul, B., Roebuck, L., Friedman, R., McDonald, B., & Chambers, K. (1996). *Health care reform tracking project: Tracking state health care reforms as they affect children and adolescents with emotional disorders and their families. 1995 state survey.* Tampa: University of South Florida, Florida Mental Health Institute.

Ridgely, M. S., Giard, J., & Shern, D. (1999). Florida's Medicaid mental health carve-out: Lessons from the first years of implementation. *Journal of Behavioral Health Services and Research, 26,* 400–415.

Stroul, B. (1996a). Introduction: Progress in children's mental health. In B. A. Stroul (Ed.), *Children's mental health: Creating systems of care in a changing society* (pp. xxi–xxxii). Baltimore: Brookes.

Stroul, B. (1996b). *Managed care and children's mental health. Proceedings of the May 1995 state managed care meeting.* Washington, DC: Georgetown University Child Development Center, National Technical Assistance Center for Children's Mental Health.

Stroul, B., & Friedman, R. (1986). *A system of care for children & youth with severe emotional disturbances* (Rev. ed.). Washington, DC: Georgetown University Child Development Center, CASSP Technical Assistance Center.

Stroul, B., Pires, S., & Armstrong, M. (1998a). *Evaluation of the Comprehensive Community Mental Health Services for Children and Their Families Program: Special study on managed care.* Atlanta, GA: Macro International, Inc.

Stroul, B., Pires, S., & Armstrong, M. (1998b). *Health care reform tracking project: Tracking state health care reforms as they affect children and adolescents with emotional disorders and their families—1997 Impact Analysis.* Tampa: University of South Florida, Florida Mental Health Institute.

Stroul, B. A., Pires, S. A., & Armstrong, M. I. (in press). *Health care reform tracking project: Tracking state health care reforms as they affect children and adolescents with behavioral health disorders and their families—2000 State Survey.* Tampa: University of South Florida, Louis de la Parte Florida Mental Health Institute, Department of Child and Family Studies, Research and Training Center for Children's Mental Health.

Stroul, B., Pires, S., Roebuck, L., Friedman, R., Barrett, B., Chambers, K., & Kershaw, M. A. (1997). State health care reforms: How they affect children and adolescents with emotional disorders and their families. *Journal of Mental Health Services and Administration, 24,* 585–598.

U.S. General Accounting Office. (1995). *Medicaid: Spending pressures drive states toward program reinvention* (GAO Rep. No. HEHS-95-122). Gaithersburg, MD: Author.

Yin, R. (1984). Case study research: Design and methods (Rev. ed.). *Applied social research methods series, volume 5* (pp. 13–26). Thousand Oaks, CA: Sage.

CHILDREN'S SERVICES: SOCIAL POLICY, RESEARCH, AND PRACTICE, 5(1), 37–56
Copyright © 2002, Lawrence Erlbaum Associates, Inc.

System-of-Care Assessment: Cross-Site Comparison of Findings

Ana Maria Brannan and Lela N. Baughman
ORC Macro
Atlanta, GA

Erika D. Reed
Westat
Atlanta, GA

Judith Katz-Leavy
Center for Mental Health Services
Rockville, MD

In this article we describe a system-level assessment that examined the extent to which 8 system-of-care principles (e.g., family-focused care, coordination of services, use of least restrictive service options) were operationalized across 8 system components (e.g., system governance, quality monitoring, case monitoring and review). Data were collected in 3 federally funded systems of care and 3 matched comparison sites. Comparisons of system scores across paired sites suggested that the federal program that funded the systems of care helped those sites come closer than the comparison sites to the ideals articulated in the principles. There was also less variability in scores across the funded systems of care, with greater variability found across the comparison sites' scores. Some movement toward the system-of-care approach was demonstrated in the comparison sites, however, despite their lack of special funding. The systems of care performed especially well in the principles of interagency involvement and community-based service delivery. Although they generally performed better than the comparison sites, the systems of care continued to struggle in their system-level quality improvement efforts and in culturally competent service delivery.

Requests for reprints should be sent to Ana Maria Brannan, ORC Macro, 3 Corporate Square, Suite 370, Atlanta, GA 30329. E-mail: abrannan@macroint.com

Since 1993, the Center for Mental Health Services (CMHS) of the Substance Abuse and Mental Health Services Administration (SAMHSA) of the U.S. Department of Health and Human Services has funded the Comprehensive Community Mental Health Services for Children and Their Families Program. This program has provided grants to 67 municipal, county, and state governments to develop systems of care in local communities. Utilizing the system-of-care approach (CMHS, 1998, in review-a, in review-b; Holden, Friedman, & Santiago, 2001; Stroul & Friedman, 1986), communities have used these funds to develop interagency linkages, strengthen family advocacy activities, broaden service arrays, enhance case management services, expand training activities, and engage in other system-of-care development efforts. This national program also funded an evaluation that included several quasi-experimental comparison studies to test the effectiveness of CMHS-funded systems of care (hereafter referred to as the comparison study). In the first phase of the evaluation, the comparison study included three communities funded in 1993 and 1994 to develop systems of care and three matched comparison sites that had not received such funding.

The underlying assumption of the system-of-care theory is that a fully implemented system of care will lead to more effective service delivery, improved clinical and functional outcomes, and greater satisfaction with services (CMHS, 1998, in review-a, in review-b; Stroul & Friedman, 1986). Key to testing this theory is determining the extent to which a true system of care is actually operating in the funded communities. It is also important to document whether elements of the system-of-care approach have emerged in the comparison communities, despite their lack of funding. Documenting system development in funded and nonfunded communities is a primary task in this comparison study and the goal of the study reported here.

The term *system of care* emerged in the early to mid-1980s to represent a cohesive network of entities from various service sectors working together to meet the total needs of children with special needs and their families (Knitzer, 1982; Stroul & Friedman, 1986). This call was based on ample evidence that many children need services from various sectors and that the linkages among sectors to enable a system of care to perform effectively were inadequate or nonexistent.

The system-of-care approach was designed to address the individual needs of children with emotional and behavioral disorders and their families and called for delivery systems and service providers to embrace articulated principles of care (Stroul & Friedman, 1986). A key feature of a system of care is the integration and coordination of all child-serving sectors including mental health, education, child welfare, juvenile justice, and (physical) health care sectors. Within each of these sectors, smaller systems operate that embody the principles, values, and goals of the larger cross-sector system. The mental health system of care offers a wide array of formal services including crisis stabilization, outpatient therapy, inpatient hospitalization, day treatment, therapeutic group and foster homes, after-school programs, and family support services such as respite care (Stroul & Friedman, 1986). In addition, the system emphasizes treating children using the least restrictive service options and keeping children with their families and in their own communities whenever possible. With the help of a case management mechanism, children move through services more efficiently, in accordance with the children's changing therapeutic needs.

Over the past 15 years, systems of care have been broadly promoted to improve delivery of mental health and support services to children with emotional and behavioral problems and their families (Davis, Yelton, Katz-Leavy, & Lourie, 1995; England & Cole, 1998; Farmer, 2000; Holden et al., 2001; Illback & Neill, 1995). Research at the system level has become increasingly important as various reform efforts manipulate resources and organizational relationships (Brown et al., 1994; Shaw, 1995). Observers have also stressed the importance of studying the relation among those sectors and among organizations within sectors (Burns & Friedman, 1990; Heflinger & Northrup, 1998; Morrissey, Johnsen, & Calloway, 1998; Sondheimer & Evans, 1995).

In this article we describe findings from an assessment of six mental health systems. This study defines the mental health system as the network of mental health service agencies, as well as public and private providers, present in the mental health sector within a community. The mental health system level includes factors such as the range of mental health services available; the organizational and financial arrangements that characterize the relationships among clients, services, and payers; the identified target population; and the system's overarching values and goals (Burns & Friedman, 1990).

METHOD

This study was conducted in the context of a quasi-experimental comparison study designed to test the effectiveness of systems of care, funded through the Comprehensive Community Mental Health Services for Children and Their Families Program, compared to traditional systems without this funding mechanism. In addition to the system-level assessment described here, the comparison study included several other evaluation components including an outcome study, a practice-level study (Hernandez et al., 2001), and a services and costs study. Three CMHS-funded systems of care, that initially received service grants in 1993 and 1994, participated in the study. These sites were selected from among the grantee sites that scored in the top quartile on an earlier system assessment instrument (Vinson, Brannan, Baughman, Wilce, & Gawron, 2001). Three comparison communities were chosen that matched their system-of-care counterparts in terms of community demographics (e.g., population size, child age distributions, racial and ethnic composition), geographic information (e.g., size of catchment area, urban or rural), and economics of the community (e.g., per capita income, proportion of families living below the poverty level). Service system characteristics were also considered, including the rate at which children were enrolled in mental health services and referral patterns. Table 1 lists the location of the systems of care and their comparison sites. For two of the pairs, it was possible to find comparison sites in the same state. For the system of care located in California, however, an out-of-state comparison site was found because California has legislated statewide implementation of systems of care, making it impossible to find an adequate comparison site in that state.

Sample

The unit of analysis for this study was the service system. All six systems (i.e., the three funded systems of care and three comparison sites) were assessed. For the three funded systems of care, the assessment focused on the last year of their 5-year funding period. It is important to note that one of the comparison sites, Austin, Texas, was funded by the program after data collection for the comparison study had begun. Although the assessment covered the year before funding, it is likely that some of the infrastructure development had already begun during the assessment period as the site prepared for their grant application submission. In particular, the grant application required articulated commitments from family organizations and core child-serving agencies, and sites were funded, in part, on the extent to which those relations had already developed.

Bounding the system in each of the comparison study communities presented challenges. Because the overall goal of the comparison study was to compare outcomes of children served in funded and nonfunded communities, the boundaries were defined in terms of the system that served the children and families who were recruited into the outcome study component of the comparison study. This led to different system definitions for each pair. In the Ohio communities, children and families were recruited into the outcome component of the comparison study through community mental health centers. Hence, in those sites, bounding the system began at those centers and radiated outward to the public agencies, family organizations, and ancillary service providers within that catchment area. In another pair, Santa Cruz, California, and Austin (i.e., Travis County), Texas were both

TABLE 1
Comparison Study Pairs and Their Locations

Comparison Study Pair	Funded System of Care	Matched Comparison
Pair 1	Stark County, Ohio	Mahoning County, Ohio
Pair 2	East Baltimore, Maryland	West Baltimore, Maryland
Pair 3	Santa Cruz, California	Austin, Texas

county-based systems, and children and families were recruited into the outcome study from county-sponsored agencies. These systems were, therefore, bounded largely along county lines, and administrators and staff were interviewed who served in parallel positions in each county.

The Baltimore pair presented a special challenge. The system of care there comprised one census tract in a disadvantaged neighborhood in East Baltimore. Children and families were recruited into the outcome component of the comparison study through the single point of entry of the system of care. To parallel that process in West Baltimore, children were recruited through the same public agencies that served as referral sources into the East Baltimore system of care (i.e., schools, juvenile justice, child welfare, and mental health). To identify appropriate respondents in West Baltimore, every effort was made to interview individuals in public agencies parallel to those interviewed in East Baltimore. In addition, considerable effort was made to locate any governing bodies, family organizations, or tertiary case review structures that had the potential to shape the system that served the children and families participating in the larger comparison study.

In each site, approximately 30 system participants were interviewed about their experiences with the mental health system in their community. Respondents included top administrators (e.g., directors of funded projects, executive directors of the community mental health centers, county administrators), family advocates, direct service providers, intake staff, representatives of child-serving agencies, quality monitoring or evaluation staff, members of tertiary case review bodies, and caregivers (e.g., parents) of children served in the system.

Measure

To assess the extent to which the funded and comparison communities embodied the system-of-care principles in their routine operations, a system-level assessment instrument was developed. The system-level assessment included qualitative methods to describe the approaches used by grantee communities to implement system-of-care principles and quantitative ratings of the extent to which system-of-care principles were achieved within each community.

The development of this system assessment instrument began with an overarching conceptual framework. The framework was organized into two domains. The system infrastructure domain was defined as the organizational arrangements and procedural framework that support and facilitate service delivery. The service delivery domain was comprised of the activities and processes undertaken to provide services directly to children and families for the purpose of treating mental, emotional, and behavioral disorders experienced by children and to support families caring for children with emotional and behavioral disorders.

For each domain, four generic components were identified that can be found in most service systems. In the system infrastructure domain, the components were governance, management and operations, service array, and quality monitoring. The components of the service delivery domain included entry into the service system, service planning, service provision, and care monitoring (see Table 2 for definitions of system components). Eight system-of-care principles were selected for assessment, including the following: family focused, individualized, culturally competent, interagency, community based, accessible, coordinated and collaborative, and least restrictive (see Table 3 for definitions of principles). This framework was organized into a matrix with system components as the columns, and the principles making up the rows. Implicit in this framework is the belief that system-of-care principles should infuse virtually all components of the system.

TABLE 2
Definitions of System Components

Domain	Definition
Infrastructure	
Governance	The governing structure responsible for explicating the system's goals, vision, and mission; strategic planning and policy development; and establishing formal arrangements among agencies. This structure may include boards of directors, oversight or steering committees, and interagency boards.
Management and operations	The administrative functions and activities that support direct service delivery. This framework focuses primarily on staff development, funding approaches, and procedural mechanisms related to the implementation of the service system.
Service array	The range of service and support options available to children and their families through the system.
Quality monitoring	Quality management throughout the system conducted through the grievance procedure, the integration of process assessment and outcome measurement, and the use of continuous feedback loops to improve service delivery.
Service delivery	
Entry	The processes and activities associated with the child's and family's initial contact with the service system(s), including the referral process and eligibility determination.
Service planning	The identification of services for the child and family through an initial process and periodic updating of service plans.
Service provision	The processes and activities related to the child's and family's ongoing receipt of and participation in services.
Care monitoring and review	Processes and activities to assess and reassess service delivery, including monitoring of the care provided to individual children and families. Processes also include review of the care of individual children to address complex issues and challenging problems to prevent the use of more restrictive services.

TABLE 3
Definitions of System-of-Care Principles

Principle	Definition
Family focused	The recognition that (a) the ecological context of the family is central to the care of all children; (b) families are important contributors to, and equal partners in, any effort to serve children; and (c) all system and service processes should maximize family involvement and address family needs.
Culturally competent	Sensitivity and responsiveness to, and acknowledgment of, the inherent value of differences related to race, religion, language, national origin, gender, socioeconomic background, and community-specific characteristics.
Interagency	The involvement and partnership of core agencies in multiple child-serving sectors, including child welfare, health, juvenile justice, education, and mental health.
Community based	The provision of services within close geographical proximity to the targeted community.
Accessible	The minimizing of barriers to services in terms of physical location, convenience of scheduling, and financial constraints.
Coordination and collaboration	Professionals working together in a complementary manner to avoid duplication of services, eliminate gaps in care, and facilitate the child's and family's movement through the service system.
Individualized	The provision of care that is expressly child centered, addresses the child's specific needs, and recognizes and incorporates the child's strengths.
Least restrictive	The priority that services should be delivered in settings that maximize freedom of choice and movement and present opportunities to interact in normative environments (e.g., school and family).

For each cell where the components and principles intersect, key indicators were identified. These indicators represented the structures or activities that would be present if a given system component did indeed realize a given principle. In developing indicators, actual behavior was prioritized over verbal commitments, future plans, or articulated ideas. For example, in the cell that intersects the service planning component and the accessibility principle, the following indicators were listed:

- Service planning occurs at flexible times to maximize the convenience for the child and family.
- Service planning occurs at a variety of places to maximize the convenience for the child and family.
- The service plan is fully accessible to families.

Through the development process, including expert review and pilot-testing, indicators were favored that could be measured well with the data collection options available. As a result, the number of indicators varied across cells ranging from 0 to 4 indicators per cell. Ultimately, 101 scoreable indicators remained in the framework across 51 of the original 64 cells.

The system assessment data collection tools were developed following this framework. Through this process, 11 semistructured interviews were developed to collect information from a variety of individuals (e.g., administrators, family members, direct service providers) involved with system development and service delivery in the assessed communities. When possible, multiple respondents were asked about the same indicators. For example, questions about the service planning indicators listed previously were asked of caregivers and case managers. The semistructured interviews varied in length requiring 30 min (e.g., for the intake worker) to 2 hr (e.g., for the project director) to complete. Some of the items in the interviews were included for context or descriptive purposes, whereas others link to indicators in the framework.

For the interview questions that mapped to framework indicators, interviewers rated the item using the response provided by the individual respondent. Explicit criteria were developed for rating each item; that is, the qualitative data collected in the semistructured interviews were used to rate each response. The responses of the various informants were rated separately, and information obtained from other sources could not be used to score an individual informant's response.

The interview items that mapped to indicators were rated on a 4-point scale, ranging from 1 (*lowest*) to 4 (*highest*). For most items, a score of 1 indicated that the site had made no effort toward implementing that indicator, and a score of 2 indicated that although some effort may have been made in this area, it was minimally effective in accomplishing the intended goal. This might be the case if the site had just begun to put a procedure in place, but it was not yet fully implemented and little or no benefit had yet been realized. A score of 3 suggested that efforts were in place and considered somewhat effective but more could be done to fully implement the principle. A score of 4 indicated that efforts were fully implemented, had been very effective in accomplishing that principle, and that little or no improvement was necessary. For other items, the 1 to 4 scale was a count. For example, several items asked how many child-serving agencies were involved in a given activity such as participation in governing bodies, quality monitoring, or service planning.

In addition to the interviews, four forms were developed to help the communities provide additional information about the composition of their governing bodies, range of their service array, staff positions funded through the grant, budgets, and participants in any tertiary case review bodies.

Measurement quality.   In the development process, several steps were taken to maximize measurement quality. First, the framework and its indicators were informed by the experience gained from previously conducted annual site visits to over 22 communities who had also received CMHS funding to develop systems of care (Vinson et al., 2001). Second, the framework and its indicators were reviewed by experts in the field to ensure content validity. Revisions were made based on expert feedback. Third, the interviews were developed following closely from the revised framework indicators. Fourth, the interviews were pilot-tested in four grantee communities not involved in the comparison study; revisions were made based on those experiences. Nearly final versions of key interviews were then reviewed by experts, and final revisions were made.

Because the system-level assessment was designed to track system development over time and to compare across systems, it was imperative that the quantitative ratings be reliable. Of particular concern was interrater reliability; that is, the extent to which different raters using the same information to rate a site would generate the same score. During development and throughout the pilot-testing process, interrater reliability was assessed among the three persons most closely involved in the development process. Rating criteria for each item was made as explicit as possible to reduce variation across raters, and site visitors were trained to apply those criteria in a standard fashion. Moreover, each site visitor was required to achieve 85% agreement with the correct ratings for 25 hypothetical interview scripts. Field assessments of interrater reliability were also conducted with one rater leading an interview and both recording information; both raters scored the interview independently. Agreement on item ratings among the pairs of raters who conducted the site visits for this study ranged from 84% to 92% in field assessments.

Data Collection

The data collection process began with a review of documents and completed forms provided by the communities. The bulk of the data collection occurred during a 3-day site visit during which system-of-care participants were interviewed. Finally, randomly selected case records were reviewed. These data were collected at the end of the funding period for the funded systems of care. Comparison sites were assessed within 3 months of the system of care. The same pair of raters assessed both sites for each comparison pair (i.e., the funded and the comparison site).

ANALYSIS

As the unit of analysis is the system, the sample size ($N = 6$) was too small for traditional statistical tests. Instead, information was presented in a descriptive fashion, highlighting differences and similarities between the funded and the comparison service systems. As the system assessment utilized a mixed method approach, both quantitative and qualitative data were reported. Specifically, quantitative scores were summarized, and qualitative information was used to provide a context for the summary scores.

Regarding the quantitative data, two summary scores were presented: mean cell scores and aggregate scores for each principle within each of the two domains. Mean cell scores were computed as the average of all scored item responses for all indicators in that cell. For example, if there were three indicators in the cell and each indicator was made up of items from six respondents (e.g., three caregivers and three case managers), then the cell mean score was the average of the 18 items (i.e., three caregiver responses per indicator, plus three case manager responses per indicator, times three indicators). Mean principle scores were computed for each domain by averaging all the scored responses across all respondents across all indicators in the cells. Qualitative data were derived from the interview responses, documentation that system administrators provided, and case record reviews. Qualitative data were reviewed to describe the differences and similarities across systems identified through the quantitative scores.

RESULTS

Tables 4 and 5 present the mean cell scores for the infrastructure and service delivery domains, respectively, and compare the overall mean scores for the funded systems of care and the comparison communities. Several general observations can be made from these data. The means tend to be higher than originally expected, with many means above the score of 2 (i.e., on a 1 to 4 scale). For both systems of care and comparison sites, scores were higher in the service delivery domain than in the infrastructure domain, suggesting that changing systems may be more difficult than changing individual practice. The funded systems of care tended to perform best on the principles of interagency involvement in the infrastructure domain and community-based service delivery in the service delivery domain. The comparison sites tended to score best on accessibility in the infrastructure domain, with no trend emerging in the service delivery domain. The funded systems performed less well in quality monitoring across principles but still received scores above those of the comparison sites, for the most part.

The scores for the systems of care were generally higher than those received by the comparison sites. In the systems of care, for example, no means were below 2, and 75% (i.e., 39 of 52) of means were above 3.0. In contrast, 23% (i.e., 13 of 52) of the comparison sites' cell scores were below 2, and 23% (i.e., 12 of 53) were above 3. The systems of care scored higher, on average, than the comparison sites

TABLE 4
Infrastructure Domain: Comparison of Descriptive Statistics on Cell Scores

| | Governance | | | | Management and Operations | | | | Service Array | | | | Quality Monitoring | | | |
| | SOC | | Comp | | SOC | | Comp | | SOC | | Comp | | SOC | | Comp | |
Principle	M	SD	M	SD	M	SD	M	SD	M	SD	M	SD	M	SD	M	SD
Family focused	2.62	1.44	2.56	1.50	2.97	0.29	1.42	0.42	—	—	—	—	2.72	0.21	2.07	0.46
Individualized	—	—	—	—	3.08	0.59	1.47	0.24	3.24	0.44	2.58	0.63	3.09	0.83	1.75	0.35
Culturally competent	—	—	—	—	3.00	0.00	2.00	1.00	2.44	1.30	1.83	0.76	3.75	0.35	2.25	0.35
Interagency	3.78	0.01	1.92	1.59	3.83	0.29	1.44	0.01	—	—	—	—	3.75	0.35	1.75	0.35
Community based	—	—	—	—	—	—	—	—	3.61	0.35	1.93	1.20	3.50	0.71	2.17	1.00
Accessible	3.64	0.32	2.85	1.6	3.72	0.25	3.50	0.50	3.74	0.13	3.03	0.45	2.50	0.21	2.00	1.40
Coordinated	3.05	0.63	2.06	1.40	3.33	0.58	2.56	0.77	3.83	0.29	2.33	1.20	2.50	2.10	2.50	2.10
Least restrictive	—	—	—	—	3.28	0.25	2.50	0.50	—	—	—	—	2.50	1.10	1.00	0.00

Note. Cells with no scoreable indicators are indicated with a dash. SOC = system of care; Comp = comparison.

TABLE 5
Service Delivery Domain: Comparison of Descriptive Statistics on Cell Scores

System Components in the Service Delivery Domain

Principle	Entry				Service Planning				Service Provision				Care Review and Monitoring			
	SOC		Comp		SOC		Comp		SOC		Comp		SOC		Comp	
	M	SD	M	SD	M	SD	M	SD	M	SD	M	SD	M	SD	M	SD
Family focused	3.83	.29	3.78	.39	3.24	.18	2.19	.39	3.33	.13	2.67	.58	3.45	.31	2.75	.33
Individualized	—	—	—	—	3.07	.33	2.41	.16	3.51	.22	3.35	.01	3.60	.24	2.92	.14
Culturally competent	3.50	.50	1.56	.51	2.38	.73	1.67	.88	2.43	.78	2.67	.88	2.73	1.1	3.33	.58
Interagency	3.78	.20	2.50	1.5	3.17	.67	1.62	.40	—	—	—	—	3.57	.50	3.67	.58
Community based	—	—	—	—	3.67	.58	2.67	.57	4.00	.00	3.52	.50	3.67	.58	2.57	.87
Accessible	3.48	.50	3.40	.11	3.60	.01	2.78	.35	3.54	.20	3.14	.14	2.11	1.3	1.08	.14
Coordinated	3.17	.76	3.33	.29	2.88	.33	2.26	.56	3.63	.23	2.76	.32	3.67	.58	2.5	1.3
Least restrictive	—	—	—	—	—	—	—	—	3.67	.58	3.0	.5	3.3	.58	3.0	.00

Note. Cells with no scoreable indicators are indicated with a dash. SOC = System of care; Comp = comparison.

in 47 of the 52 cells, with the comparison sites scoring the same or slightly higher than the systems of care in only 5 cells.

Another general observation was that there was less variability in cell scores across the systems of care than across the comparison sites. This was indicated by the considerably smaller standard deviations in the scores for the systems of care than for the comparison sites, especially in the infrastructure domain. This lack of variability suggests that CMHS funding helped those communities embody system-of-care principles at similar levels. The variability found in the comparison sites' scores suggests that, although individual sites experienced some success in certain areas, they were generally more inconsistent in their application of system-of-care principles than were the funded systems of care.

Although the mean cell scores provide an overall comparison of system-of-care sites to the comparison sites, examination of differences in the matched pairs is more meaningful. Figures 1 through 3 present the overall principle scores by domain, across system components.

In Figure 1, Ohio's Stark and Mahoning Counties are compared. Stark County, the funded system of care, received higher scores on all principles except (a) accessibility of services at the infrastructure level and (b) least restrictive care at the service delivery level. These differences were more dramatic in the infrastructure domain, especially for the principles of individualized care, interagency involvement, and coordinated service delivery. Although both communities did well in terms of accessibility of services, Mahoning county's higher score within the infra-

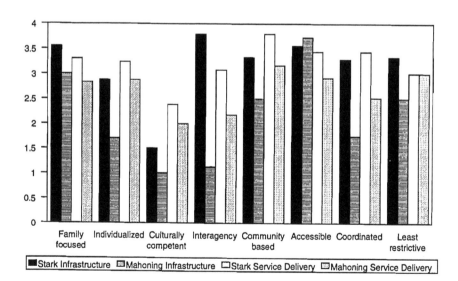

FIGURE 1   Ohio pair: Comparison of overall principle scores by domain.

structure domain can be explained primarily by that sites' quality monitoring efforts to identify and correct access problems for their clients at the mental health center (e.g., adjusting the hours that the psychiatrist was available based on findings from a client satisfaction survey). Both sites had multiple satellite offices and provided services in schools; however, providers in Stark County were much more likely to conduct home visits. This explains, in part, why Stark County earned a higher score for accessibility in the service delivery domain.

In the service delivery domain, the greatest differences were in the principles of interagency involvement, community-based care, and coordinated service delivery. Although scores for least restrictive care in the infrastructure domain were higher in Stark County, the two communities received identical scores for this area in the service delivery domain. This was due to similar case review structures, present in both sites, that reviewed all requests for publicly funded residential treatment and that the state of Ohio encouraged all counties to establish. Although the case review structure in Stark County was reportedly more family focused, with more interagency involvement, and better coordination of care, the structures in both counties were similarly effective in preventing residential placement.

The Baltimore pair is compared in Figure 2. In this pair, the funded system of care scored higher than the comparison pair for each principle in both domains. As with the Ohio pair, the differences between the scores were typically greater in the infrastructure domain. The areas of greatest difference in that domain were family focus, cultural competence, and interagency involvement. Family members in the

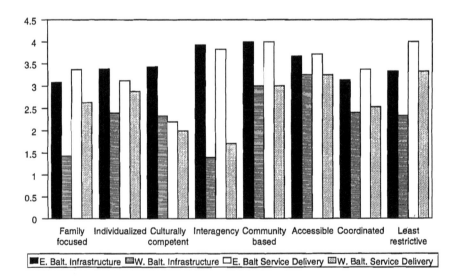

FIGURE 2   Baltimore pair: Comparison of overall principle scores by domain.

East Baltimore system of care were actively involved in the system's governing body (e.g., formulating policy, developing the service array), management and operations (e.g., staff recruitment, staff training, holding staff positions), and quality monitoring efforts (e.g., collecting data, initiating special studies). In the West Baltimore site, virtually no family involvement was reported at the system level.

East Baltimore had the highest cultural competence score in the infrastructure domain of any of the sites assessed. This site drew on members of the community to provide support services (i.e., neighborhood liaisons), to recruit clinicians and staff who reflected the cultural make-up of the children and families served, and to provide cultural competence training to staff of other community programs.

There was considerable difference between the Baltimore sites in the interagency principle. The funded East Baltimore system of care received a nearly perfect score for having active involvement of all the child-serving sectors (i.e., mental health, juvenile justice, education, social services, and child welfare) in system governance at the upper and middle management levels. This site also integrated line staff across agencies and sectors by conducting joint training, sharing staff positions (i.e., cofunded by two agencies), and out-stationing staff from the funded grant project to other agency offices. A particular strength of this site was the involvement of multiple agencies in quality monitoring efforts including the development of an instrument to assess interagency collaboration. In contrast, although interviews were conducted with staff from education, juvenile justice, child welfare, and mental health, respondents from the West Baltimore agencies reported virtually no interaction across agencies.

The differences in the service delivery domain scores were greatest for the principles of interagency involvement, community-based care, and coordinated service delivery. At the service delivery level, interagency involvement at the East Baltimore site was achieved through the active involvement of all child-serving agencies in the intake process (i.e., all agencies could initiate enrollment of children into the grant-funded system), routine multi-agency participation in the development and monitoring of individual service plans, and the involvement of multiple agencies in the tertiary case review body. The East Baltimore site also received the highest possible score for the community-based principle largely because of its emphasis on providing a full range of services within the immediate community, and the routine provision of services in families' homes. In addition, innovative and support services and flexible funding were used to create alternatives to out-of-home and out-of-community placements. These included emergency respite services, intensive home-based services, and afterschool programs. Strong interagency involvement facilitated coordination and collaboration of service delivery in the East Baltimore system across a variety of agencies and community service providers. This was evident in the process for service planning, service provision, monitoring of care, and child and family transitions across services.

The overall principle scores for the Santa Cruz and Austin pair are presented in Figure 3. Austin, the comparison site, performed better than the funded Santa Cruz system of care on the principle of family focus in the infrastructure domain, although neither site excelled in this area. The Santa Cruz system had two official slots for family members on their governing body; however, no family member had attended the meetings held in the assessment year, limiting family representation in system governance. There was a family advisory council with family representation, but this body did not perform governing functions. In addition, families were involved only minimally in quality monitoring efforts. Austin had only one family representative on the governing body (out of 13 members), and respondents reported that not all members were receptive to the family representative's input.

The Santa Cruz system received higher scores for the remainder of the principles. The greatest differences in the infrastructure domain were for the principles of individualized care, community-based service delivery, and use of least restrictive service options. The difference in the individualized care scores were primarily due to Santa Cruz's structured multidisciplinary team approach to service delivery, the use of paraprofessionals to provide a variety of unique services, and the availability of a wide range of services to build on children's strengths (e.g., poetry, art and karate classes, climbing clubs). The difference in scores for the community-based and least restrictive principles in the infrastructure domain can be explained by the presence, in Santa Cruz, of intermediate service and support options that were used to encourage the use of least restrictive settings and to avert

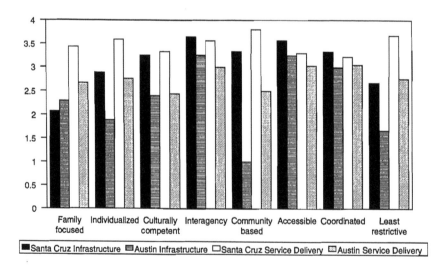

FIGURE 3   Santa Cruz and Austin pair: Comparison of overall principle scores by domain.

out-of-community placements. Note, however, that Santa Cruz's score on least restrictiveness, although higher than Austin's, was just above the midpoint indicating that this was not a great strength for that site. This score was due primarily to the absence of evaluation efforts (e.g., routine and systematic collection and analysis of data) to inform system quality improvement in the area of least restrictive service delivery.

The Austin site's lower scores on both individualized care and community-based service delivery were related to the limited service array and insufficient service capacity at the time in the assessment period. The lack of intermediate service options and support services, as well as long waits for services, reportedly compromised that site's ability to individualize care for children and required a substantial minority of children to leave the community for several types of services.

In the service delivery domain, the greatest differences in scores were for cultural competence, community-based, and least restrictive care. Both sites included large Hispanic communities, and both sites made efforts to address the cultural needs of this population. In both sites, intake, service planning, and service provision could be conducted in Spanish, although difficulty hiring enough bilingual staff and clinicians was reported in both sites. The Santa Cruz site, however, conducted more outreach to minority communities and directly addressed families' cultural preferences in their service planning process.

The community-based and least restrictive care scores in the service delivery domain for both sites were higher than those found in the infrastructure domain, and the magnitude of the differences between sites was somewhat smaller. Santa Cruz's higher scores were due primarily to an emphasis on using community-based options and least restrictive settings throughout the process of planning and providing services. In addition, a central database was used to help agencies work together to monitor individual placements, service episodes, and costs of care. Respondents in Austin reported that there were no formal mechanisms in place to monitor the care of children receiving services outside the community, or to plan their return.

DISCUSSION

In general, the funded systems embodied system-of-care principles to a greater extent than did their matched comparison sites. In addition, performance on this assessment was more consistent among funded sites than among comparison sites. In particular, the funding appeared to bolster infrastructure development especially for interagency involvement and community-based care. The differences between funded and comparison systems were smaller in magnitude for the service delivery domain. However, in the service delivery domain, each funded system of care performed better than its matched comparison sites in the areas of community-based and least restrictive care. This provides some support for the position that expanding the array of service options available in the community reduces the use of residential services.

Despite the additional funding, however, there were some areas in which the systems of care continued to struggle. The systems of care performed less well in quality monitoring than any other system components. This assessment focused on the routine collection, analysis and use of data to identify and resolve problems in the system at the aggregate level. Although most sites conducted quality-monitoring efforts at the individual level (e.g., peer review of records), few aggregated data to examine broader trends across the system. The federal grant required sites to participate in evaluation efforts and provided funds for that purpose. However, respondents were typically unable to describe how the data collected under the requirements of the grant were used to inform system improvements. In addition, the funded systems of care did not fully incorporate cultural competence in routine practice, with few examples given of moving beyond providing cultural competence training. This is consistent with earlier findings (Vinson et al., 2001), suggesting that operationalizing this principle presents special challenges. Family involvement in system governance was a distinguishing feature in only the Baltimore pair, primarily because families were so poorly represented in West Baltimore at the system level.

It is noteworthy that, even without additional funding, the comparison sites were making some strides toward realizing system-of-care principles, especially in terms of accessibility of services. The language of systems of care and the value of the principles were present in all the comparison communities and mentioned by many of the respondents. Without funding, however, it appeared that the execution of those principles lagged behind.

Several limitations to this study warrant mentioning. The greatest of these is the difficulty inherent in truly capturing the complexities of a mental health service delivery system using responses from approximately 30 individuals. Several features of the assessment protect against this limitation including the careful selection of respondents, the comprehensiveness of the information collected on each site, and the reliance on participants to inform the areas most familiar to them (e.g., asking direct service providers about their routine practice and not about system governance issues). Another concern is that the site visitors who interviewed participants and rated their responses were aware of which sites were the funded systems of care and which were the comparison sites (i.e., they could not be kept "blind" to condition). The emphasis on adherence to criteria, however, likely served to minimize the risk of bias in scoring that may have otherwise resulted.

The field of mental health services research has before it the difficult challenge of assessing the implementation of efforts to develop systems of care and interpret the impact of those changes on mental health service utilization and outcomes.

Perhaps the primary task is to distinguish between service-level efforts to coordinate and deliver services to individual clients and attempts to achieve broader organizational coordination across sectors. Until this distinction is clearly articulated, service integration will likely remain the responsibility of individual case managers, treatment teams, or programs, precluding the long-lasting changes to organizational structures that can bolster the efforts of individual providers of services. It may never be possible to assess the unique effects of changes at the system-level on mental health service use because a multitude of child-, provider-, and community-level factors will also likely be involved. However, the potential to improve service delivery through improvements at the system-level is great, as relationships at this level are likely to influence factors and relationships at other levels.

ACKNOWLEDGMENTS

Development of this assessment tool and collection of these data were supported by the Center for Mental Health Services, Substance Abuse and Mental Health Services Administration, United States Department of Health and Human Services (Contract Numbers 280–97–8014, 280–99–8023, and 280–00–8040).

We thank the administrators, service providers, and families who participated in this study.

REFERENCES

Brown, L., Cox, G. B., Jones, W. E., Semke, J., Allen, D. G., Gilchrist, L. D., & Sutphen-Mroz, J. (1994). Effects of mental health reform on client characteristics, continuity of care and community tenure. *Evaluation and Program Planning, 17,* 63–72.

Burns, B. J., & Friedman, R. M. (1990). Examining the research base for child mental health services and policy. *Journal of Mental Health Administration, 17,* 87–98.

Center for Mental Health Services. (1998). *Annual report to Congress on the evaluation of the Comprehensive Community Mental Health Services for Children and Their Families Program, 1998.* Atlanta, GA: ORC Macro.

Center for Mental Health Services. (in review-a). *Annual report to Congress on the evaluation of the Comprehensive Community Mental Health Services for Children and Their Families Program, 1999.* Atlanta, GA: ORC Macro.

Center for Mental Health Services. (in review-b). *Annual report to Congress on the evaluation of the Comprehensive Community Mental Health Services for Children and Their Families Program, 2000.* Atlanta, GA: ORC Macro.

Davis, M., Yelton, S., Katz-Leavy, J., & Lourie, I. S. (1995). *Unclaimed Children* revisited: The status of state children's mental health service systems. *Journal of Mental Health Administration, 22,* 147–166.

England, M. J., & Cole, R. F. (1998). Preparing for communities of care for child and family mental health for the twenty-first century. *The Child Psychiatrist in the Community, 7,* 469–481.

Farmer, E. M. Z. (2000). Issues confronting effective services in systems of care. *Children and Youth Services Review, 22,* 627–650.

Heflinger, C. A., & Northrup, D. (1998). Measuring change in mental health services coordination in managed mental health care for children and adolescents. In J. P. Morrissey (Ed.), *Research in community mental health volume 9: Social networks and mental illness* (pp. 69–88). Greenwich, CT: JAI.

Hernandez, M., Gomez, A., Lipien, L., Greenbaum, P. E., Armstrong, K. H., & Gonzalez, P. (2001). Use of the system-of-care practice review in the national evaluation: Evaluating the fidelity of practice to system-of-care principles. *Journal of Emotional and Behavioral Disorders, 9,* 43–52.

Holden, E. W., Friedman, R. M., & Santiago, R. L. (2001). Overview of the National Evaluation of the Comprehensive Community Mental Health Services for Children and Their Families Program. *Journal of Emotional and Behavioral Disorders, 9,* 4–12.

Illback, R. J., & Neill, T. K. (1995). Service coordination in mental health systems for children, youth, and families: Progress, problems, prospects. *Journal of Mental Health Administration, 22,* 17–28.

Knitzer, J. (1982). *Unclaimed children.* Washington, DC: Children's Defense Fund.

Morrissey, J. P., Johnson, M. C., & Calloway, M. O. (1998). Methods for system-level evaluations of child mental health services networks. In M. H. Epstein, K. Kutash, & A. Duchnowski (Eds.), *Outcomes for children and youth with behavioral and emotional disorders and their families: Programs and evaluation best practices* (pp. 297–327). Austin, TX: PRO-ED, Inc.

Shaw, K. M. (1995). Challenges in evaluating systems reform. *The Evaluation Exchange, 1*(1), 2–3.

Sondheimer, D. L., & Evans, M. E. (1995). Developments in children's mental health services research: An overview of current and future demonstration directions. In L. Bickman & D. J. Rog (Eds.), *Children's mental health services: Policy, research, and evaluation* (pp. 64–84). Newbury Park, CA: Sage.

Stroul, B. A., & Friedman, R. M. (1986). *A system of care for children and youth with severe emotional disturbances* (Rev. ed.). Washington, DC: Georgetown University Child Development Center, CASSP Technical Assistance Center.

Vinson, N. B., Brannan, A. M., Baughman, L. B., Wilce, M., & Gawron, T. (2001). The system of care model: Implementation in 27 sites. *Journal of Emotional and Behavioral Disorders, 9,* 30–41.

CHILDREN'S SERVICES: SOCIAL POLICY, RESEARCH, AND PRACTICE, 5(1), 57–65
Copyright © 2002, Lawrence Erlbaum Associates, Inc.

Policy Implications of the National Evaluation of the Comprehensive Community Mental Health Services for Children and Their Families Program

E. Wayne Holden

ORC Macro
Atlanta, GA

Gary De Carolis

Center for Mental Health Services
Substance Abuse and Mental Health Services Administration
Rockville, MD

Barbara Huff

Federation of Families for Children's Mental Health
Alexandria, VA

The Comprehensive Community Mental Health Services for Children and Their Families Program is described. Since its inception, this program has had the goal of using federal resources to facilitate the development of community-based systems of care that will be sustained by state- and local-level resources after federal funding. Much of this work requires a sustained emphasis on the policy implications of the program to influence public policy changes. These policy implications are discussed across multiple target audiences and impact areas at the federal, state, and local levels. The professional training and research communities are highlighted as important audiences to inform to facilitate continued policy change. The relations between data from this program and other recent federal initiatives to support research and evaluation in children's mental health services are discussed.

Requests for reprints should be sent to E. Wayne Holden, ORC Macro, 3 Corporate Square, Suite 370, Atlanta, GA 30329. E-mail: wholden@macroint.com

The system-of-care approach utilized in the Comprehensive Community Mental Health Services for Children and Their Families Program has evolved into a major organizing force shaping the development of community-based children's mental health services across the United States (U.S. Department of Health and Human Services [DHHS], 1999). At its most fundamental level, this approach consists of the development of a comprehensive spectrum of mental health and other necessary services that is guided by a core set of values and guiding principles. Broadly speaking, systems of care are to be *child centered* and *family focused, community based*, and *culturally competent*. These underlying principles not only articulate the nature and quality of the services that should be provided to children and their families, but their extensions within communities establish a comprehensive model for how child-serving systems should be organized at the infrastructure level and how they should function. These principles have also become a guiding set of concepts for influencing the development and articulation of public policy that supports the improvement of community-based services for children and their families.

Providing much of the context for system-of-care development has been federal initiatives such as the 1984 Child and Adolescent Service System Program and the 1992 Comprehensive Community Mental Health Services for Children and Their Families Program (Public Health Service Act of 1992). This latter program has provided over $500 million in federal funding for the development of local systems of care, and as a result has served nearly 50,000 children and their families nationwide (Center for Mental Health Services [CMHS], 1998, in review-a, in review-b). Federal investments have not only focused on developing systems of care but also on creating change in community-based services for children that can be sustained by local-level resources. The continued support of federal funding has played a significant role in producing sustainable systems change, much of which is now being supported and replicated by local- and state-level agencies (Koyanagi & Feres-Merchant, 2000). Findings from the national evaluation of the first phase of grantees initially funded in 1993 and 1994 indicate that approaches such as cross-agency and multidisciplinary service delivery teams, shared funding of staff, and interagency planning structures are system-of-care innovations that have been accepted, promoted, and further supported by local and state resources (Vinson, Brannan, Baughman, Wilce, & Gawron, 2001). Although complicated by varying local-level circumstances and policy agendas, many of the programs that were developed by the first phase of grantees were able to achieve fiscal sustainability through such mechanisms as redirecting existing resources, pooling funds, reinvesting saved resources, and leveraging managed care (Koyanagi & Feres-Merchant, 2000; Stroul, Pires, Armstrong, & Zaro, 2002). Data on the effectiveness of services and associated costs were instrumental in mobilizing public support for sustainability efforts.

Since its inception, the Comprehensive Community Mental Health Services for Children and Their Families Program has maintained a strong evaluation component. Mandated as part of the public law that established the program (Public Health Service Act of 1992), each funded site actively participates in both national- and local-level evaluation efforts. As the program has matured, comprehensive reports of initial evaluation results have become publicly available (CMHS, 1997, 1998; Hodges, Doucette-Gates, & Kim, 2000; Hodges, Doucette-Gates, & Liao, 1999; Hodges & Kim, 2000; Holden, Friedman, & Santiago, 2001; Walrath, dosReis, et al., in press; Walrath, Mandell, & Leaf, 2001; Walrath, Mandell, et al., in press; Walrath, Sharp, Zuber, & Leaf, 2001). With data collection and evaluation of the initial 22 grantees complete, more definitive results are now emerging, particularly in the area of controlled comparison studies that were initiated later in the funding cycle in 1997 (CMHS, in review-a, in review-b; Hernandez et al., 2001; Santiago, 2001). The evaluation of 23 grantees funded initially in 1997–1998 has also begun to yield results of systems development and outcomes for individual programs (CMHS, in review-a, in review-b). This information will be complemented by results from 22 communities funded initially in 1999–2000, whose evaluation has just been initiated. These findings will contribute significantly to our collective understanding of both children's mental health and the system-of-care approach.

POLICY TARGETS AND IMPLICATIONS

The national evaluation of the Comprehensive Community Mental Health Services for Children and Their Families Program has had a goal of generating information to inform decision making at multiple levels. Within individual grantee programs, evaluation data are used to inform clinical decision making at the child and family levels and to provide data for program development. For example, grantee programs feed evaluation information back to care coordination teams so that evaluation data can be considered in ongoing care coordination and monitoring processes (A. Rosenblatt & Rosenblatt, 2000; A. Rosenblatt, Wyman, Kingdon, & Ichinose, 1998; J. A. Rosenblatt & Furlong, 1998; J. A. Rosenblatt et al., 1998; J. A. Rosenblatt & Rosenblatt, 1999; Walrath et al., 2001; Walrath, Nickerson, Crowel, & Leaf, 1998; Wood, Furlong, Casas, & Sosna, 1998). Additionally, evaluation information is used at the individual grantee level for quality monitoring purposes and to inform governance bodies who are in the position of making decisions regarding program direction (Hernandez, Hodges, & Cascardi, 1998; Wood et al., 1998; Woodbridge & Huang, 2000). What appears to be relatively simple information such as descriptive and clinical characteristics of participants at entry into services can have a profound impact on program direction when compared to community-level population data identifying those in need of services (Liao, Manteuffel,

Paulic, & Sondheimer, 2001). More complex information addressing system development across time, service costs, and outcomes for subsets of participants is obviously an important part of the outcomes accountability information feedback loop (Hernandez et al., 1998; Holden et al., 2001) that supports program development and dissemination of innovative system-of-care approaches.

Results of the national evaluation are also designed to have a significant impact on public policy regarding children's mental health services. As indicated previously, one of the chief goals of the Comprehensive Community Mental Health Services for Children and Their Families Program is to create sustainable change in infrastructure and service delivery at the community level that becomes supported by state and local sources of funding after federal investment. To that end, national evaluation data have been utilized at multiple policy levels with different target audiences.

Facilitating sustainable change in local systems of care requires impacting policy at the federal and state as well as local community levels. Multiple audiences with varying needs are the targets for such information. Audience segments at the national level such as federal agency personnel, congressmen, and national advocacy groups (e.g., Federation of Families for Children's Mental Health, National Mental Health Association) are important to inform to provide an outcomes accountability feedback loop that facilitates further national program development (Hernandez et al., 1998). Information at this level also satisfies legal obligations of the statute establishing the program to inform Congress on an annual basis, while concurrently educating decision makers about the impact of the initiative and the need for continued federal support as the impetus for community-level change. Audience segments at the state level include agency personnel and elected officials who are crafting new policy initiatives. They are particularly interested in the ability of programs to address mental health needs and impact positively on their constituents. Local-level policymakers, who are typically associated with agency administrators, are key individuals to influence. They can wield substantial influence over policies for local child serving agencies and be effective partners in sustaining the momentum necessary to produce community-level change. Finally, it is also important to disseminate evaluation data and analyses into the research community through venues such as professional conferences and the peer reviewed literature. These data can be critical in assisting researchers to develop hypotheses and questions that are more relevant to real world effectiveness than those that can be approached through small randomized clinical trials conducted with volunteer populations in university settings.

Many examples exist of policy changes facilitated by local- and national-level data within the Comprehensive Community Mental Health Services for Children and Their Families Program. From a federal perspective, evaluation data in conjunction with other systematic efforts has provided information to fuel continued growth of a program that was initially funded at $4.9 million in fiscal year 1993 and has grown to $91.7 million in fiscal year 2001. Perhaps the most compelling policy implications, however, are those changes that occur at the state and local levels that directly support the sustainability of systems of care as federal funding dissipates. For example, in the states of Rhode Island and Kansas (two grantees from the 1993–1994 cycle of funding) evaluation data documented program success to state-level policymakers that resulted in legislative changes to mandate interagency collaboration and the development of systems of care as the model for providing children's mental health services statewide. In Milwaukee, evaluation data in concert with an innovative wraparound program for juvenile offenders resulted in a special carve-out within Medicaid managed care (Stroul et al., 2002) that expanded fiscal resources for the program fourfold over the course of 2 to 3 years (Foster, Kelsch, Kamradt, Sosna, & Yang, 2001). Although in many ways more complex than other government structures, sovereign Native American tribal governments in seven funded communities are beginning to shift policy to support the further development and sustainability of systems of care (CMHS, in review-b; Cross, Earle, Echo-Hawk Solie, & Manness, 2000).

Beyond the sustainability of individual programs and dissemination of the system-of-care model at the local and state levels, implications with respect to professional training and research are also important to address. Traditional training in psychology and other related mental health fields does not provide sufficient exposure and background to the system-of-care approach. A few model programs exist nationwide, and some attention is being paid to integrating the approach into graduate-level curricula more generally (Meyers, Kaufman, & Goldman, 1999). The emphasis placed on the continued use and development of the system-of-care approach in the recent Surgeon General's Report (DHHS, 1999) indicates that more change needs to occur in the area of training for the model to disseminate fully and for professionals to be adept at its implementation without substantial retraining in the field.

Training in the area of mental health services research has also lagged behind other research approaches in professional training programs. Traditional designs used in experimental research are not directly translatable into the evaluation of complex services within community settings (Wolff, 2000). The Research and Training Centers for Children's Mental Health Services at the University of South Florida and Portland State University that are funded by the CMHS and the National Institute for Disability Determination and Research are providing more integrated approaches to services research. The former center, in particular, has embarked on an extensive 5-year research agenda to understand the development of children's mental health policy at the state and local levels. More recently, a program announcement released by the National Institute of Mental Health and the CMHS (NIMH, 2000) has established a grants program for funding services research conducted within the CMHS-funded communities that are developing systems of care. Further collaboration and integration across researchers, those involved in training mental health professionals and those individuals providing services in the field is an important component to expanding the information base to support systems of care in the future.

CONCLUSIONS

The first Surgeon General's Report on Mental Health (DHHS, 1999) provides an important context for the further development and evaluation of systems of care. The report concluded that although findings are encouraging, the effectiveness of systems of care has not been demonstrated conclusively. The Fort Bragg study (Bickman et al., 1995; Bickman, Summerfelt, & Noser, 1997) and the Stark County study (Bickman, Noser, & Summerfelt, 1999; Bickman, Summerfelt, Firth, & Douglas, 1997), in particular, did not find differential effects for broad-based continua of care, a related service system conceptual model, when outcomes were compared to matched community settings. The Surgeon General's Report indicated that further research needs to focus on the effectiveness of evidence-based services in fully integrated community settings such as those with systems of care. Furthermore, examining the relation between changes at the system level and changes at the practice level is critical. This point was also underscored by Burns, Hoagwood, and Mrazek (1999) in a comprehensive review of the literature on effectiveness of treatments for children's mental health disorders. They concluded that the relation between treatment components and the principles underlying service system delivery may be one of the most important elements influencing short- and long-term outcomes in community settings.

As noted throughout this article, the first Surgeon General's Report on Mental Health (DHHS, 1999) has been a landmark event that has provided an important baseline for measuring the progress that is made over the next decade on improving the effectiveness of children's mental health services. The report clearly details that, over the last several decades, significant resources have been devoted to and much progress has been made in developing valid and reliable diagnostic systems and testing the efficacy of treatments for specific childhood disorders under ideal conditions. Evidence from these efficacy trials indicates that treatment can have a significant positive impact on children and families when compared to groups that received no treatment, were placed on a waiting list, or were exposed to a placebo intervention. These results, however, stand in contrast to the more limited information on community-level outcomes, which provides less support for the differential effectiveness of interventions in community settings. The integration of evidence-based interventions with services in the community has become an important topic of concern, both for researchers who have developed manualized interventions and conducted efficacy trials and for those who are directly invested in developing and examining services at the community level.

The Comprehensive Community Mental Health Services for Children and Their Families Program is a potential laboratory for conducting the research necessary to understand community parameters that may facilitate or impede the effectiveness of services for children, adolescents, and their families. Results of studies conducted within these programs over the next several years can shed light on a number of community-level factors that are necessary to ensure that service systems are developed that deliver comprehensive community-based services with the highest possible fidelity. To be successful, this likely will require a stepwise approach whereby the results of smaller scale studies examining process and outcome variables from qualitative and quantitative perspectives are utilized to inform the development of larger scale, controlled investigations. The results of studies such as these combined with program evaluation data are essential to continued formation of effective public policy in the children's mental health arena (DeLeon & Williams, 1997) in the future.

ACKNOWLEDGMENTS

Work on this article was supported by contract numbers 280–97–8014, 280–99–8023, and 280–00–8040 with the Child, Adolescent and Family Branch of the Center for Mental Health Services in the federal Substance Abuse and Mental Health Services Administration, United States Department of Health and Human Services.

REFERENCES

Bickman, L., Guthrie, P. R., Foster, E. M., Lambert, W., Summerfelt, W. T., Breda, C. S., & Heflinger, C. A. (1995). *Evaluating managed mental health services: The Fort Bragg experiment.* New York: Plenum.

Bickman, L., Noser, K., & Summerfelt, W. M. (1999). Long-term effects of a system of care on children and adolescents. *The Journal of Behavioral Health Services & Research, 26,* 185–202.

Bickman, L. Summerfelt, W., Firth, J., & Douglas, S. (1997). The Stark County evaluation project: Baseline results of a randomized experiment. In C. Nixon & D. Northrup (Eds.), *Evaluating mental health services* (pp. 231–258). Thousand Oaks, CA: Sage.

Bickman, L., Summerfelt, W., & Noser, K. (1997). Comparative outcomes of emotionally disturbed children and adolescents in a system of services and usual care. *Psychiatric Services, 48,* 1543–1548.

Burns, B. J., Hoagwood, K., & Mrazek, P. J. (1999). Effective treatment for mental disorders in children and adolescents. *Clinical Child and Family Psychology Review, 2,* 199–254.

Center for Mental Health Services. (1997). *Annual report to Congress on the evaluation of the Comprehensive Community Mental Health Services for Children and Their Families Program, 1997.* Atlanta, GA: Macro International Inc.

Center for Mental Health Services. (1998). *Annual report to Congress on the evaluation of the Comprehensive Community Mental Health Services for Children and Their Families Program, 1998.* Atlanta, GA: Macro International Inc.

Center for Mental Health Services (in review-a). *Annual report to Congress on the evaluation of the Comprehensive Community Mental Health Services for Children and Their Families Program, 1999.* Atlanta, GA: ORC Macro.

Center for Mental Health Services (in review-b). *Annual report to Congress on the evaluation of the Comprehensive Community Mental Health Services for Children and Their Families Program, 2000.* Atlanta, GA: ORC Macro.

Cross, T., Earle, K., Echo-Hawk Solie, H., & Manness, K. (2000). Cultural strengths and challenges in implementing a system of care model in American Indian communities. *Systems of care: Promising practices in children's mental health, 2000 series, volume I.* Washington, DC: Center for Effective Collaboration and Practice, American Institutes for Research.

DeLeon, P. H., & Williams, J. G. (1997). Evaluation research and public policy formation: Are psychologists collectively willing to accept unpopular findings? *American Psychologist, 52,* 551–552.

Foster, E. M., Kelsch, C. C., Kamradt, B., Sosna, T., & Yang, Z. (2001). Expenditures and sustainability in systems of care. *Journal of Emotional and Behavioral Disorders, 9,* 53–62, 70.

Hernandez, M., Gomez, A., Lipien, L., Greenbaum, P. E., Armstrong, K., & Gonzalez, P. (2001). Use of the system-of-care practice review in the national evaluation: Evaluating the fidelity of practice to system-of-care principles. *Journal of Emotional and Behavioral Disorders, 9,* 43–52.

Hernandez, M., Hodges, S., & Cascardi, M. (1998). The ecology of outcomes: System accountability in children's mental health. *Journal of Behavioral Health Services & Research, 25,* 136–150.

Hodges, K., Doucette-Gates, A., & Kim, C. S. (2000). Predicting service utilization with the Child and Adolescent Functional Assessment Scale in a sample of youths with serious emotional disturbance served by Center for Mental Health Services-funded demonstrations. *Journal of Behavioral Health Services and Research, 27,* 47–59.

Hodges, K., Doucette-Gates, A., & Liao, Q. (1999). The relationship between the Child and Adolescent Functional Assessment Scale (CAFAS) and indicators of functioning. *Journal of Child and Family Studies, 8,* 109–122.

Hodges, K., & Kim, C. S. (2000). Psychometric study of the Child and Adolescent Functional Assessment Scale: Prediction of contact with the law and poor school attendance. *Journal of Abnormal Child Psychology, 28,* 287–297.

Holden, E. W., Friedman, R. M., & Santiago, R. L. (2001). Overview of the National Evaluation of the Comprehensive Community Mental Health Services for Children and Their Families Program. *Journal of Emotional and Behavioral Disorders, 9,* 4–12.

Koyanagi, C., & Feres-Merchant, D. (2000). For the long haul: Maintaining systems of care beyond the federal investment. *Systems of care: Promising practices in children's mental health, 2000 series* (Vol. 3, pp. 1–84). Washington, DC: Center for Effective Collaboration and Practice, American Institutes for Research.

Liao, Q., Manteuffel, B., Paulic, C., & Sondheimer, D. (2001). Describing the population of adolescents served in systems of care. *Journal of Emotional and Behavioral Disorders, 9,* 13–29.

Meyers, J., Kaufman, M., & Goldman, S. (1999). Promising practices: Training strategies for serving children with serious emotional disturbance and their families in a system of care. *Systems of care: Promising practices in children's mental health, 1998 series, volume V.* Washington, DC: Center for Effective Collaboration and Practice, American Institutes for Research.

National Institute of Mental Health. (2000). *Effectiveness, practice, and implementation in CMHS' children's service sites* (NIMH PA No. PA-00–135). Rockville, MD: Author.

Public Health Service Act of 1992, Pub. L. No. 102–321, as amended, § 561–565.

Rosenblatt, A., & Rosenblatt, J. A. (2000). Demographic, clinical, and functional characteristics of youth enrolled in six California systems of care. *Journal of Child and Family Studies, 9,* 51–66.

Rosenblatt, A., Wyman, N., Kingdon, D., & Ichinose, C. (1998). Managing what you measure: Creating outcome-driven systems of care for youth with severe emotional disturbances. *The Journal of Behavioral Health Services and Research, 25,* 177–203.

Rosenblatt, J. A., & Furlong, M. J. (1998). Outcomes in a system of care for youths with emotional and behavioral disorders: An examination of differential change across clinical profiles. *Journal of Child and Family Studies, 7,* 217–232.

Rosenblatt, J. A., Robertson, L. M., Bates, M. P., Wood, M., Furlong, M. J., & Sosna, T. (1998). Troubled or troubling? Characteristics of youth referred to a system of care without system-level referral constraints. *Journal of Emotional and Behavioral Disorders, 6,* 42–54.

Rosenblatt, J. A., & Rosenblatt, A. (1999). Youth functional status and academic achievement in collaborative mental health and education programs: Two California care systems. *Journal of Emotional and Behavioral Disorders, 7,* 21–30.

Santiago, R. (2001, February). *Design and methodological issues in the comparison study.* Paper presented at A System of Care for Children's Mental Heath, Expanding the Research Base: 14th Annual Research and Training Conference, Tampa, FL.

Stroul, B. A., Pires, S. A., Armstrong, M. I., & Zaro, S. (2002/this issue). The impact of managed care on systems of care that serve children with serious emotional disturbances and their families. *Children's Services: Social Policy, Research, and Practice, 5,* 21–36.

U.S. Department of Health and Human Services. (1999). *Mental Health: A Report of the Surgeon General.* Rockville, MD: U.S. Department of Health and Human Services, Substance Abuse and Mental Health Services Administration, Center for Mental Health Services, National Institutes of Health, National Institute of Mental Health.

Vinson, N., Brannan, A. M., Baughman, L., Wilce, M., & Gawron, T. (2001). The system-of-care model: Implementation in twenty-seven communities. *Journal of Emotional and Behavioral Disorders, 9,* 30–42.

Walrath, C., dosReis, S., Miech, R., Liao, Q., Holden, E. W., De Carolis, G., Santiago, R., & Leaf, P. (in press). Referral source differences in functional impairment levels for children served in the Comprehensive Community Mental Health Services for Children and Their Families Program. *Journal of Child and Family Studies.*

Walrath, C. M., Mandell, D. S., & Leaf, P. J. (2001). Responses of children with different intake profiles to mental health treatment. *Psychiatric Services, 52,* 196–201.

Walrath, C., Mandell, D., Liao, Q., Holden, E. W., De Carolis, G., Santiago, R., & Leaf, P. (in press). Suicidal behaviors among children in the Comprehensive Community Mental Health Services for Children and Their Families Program. *Journal of the American Academy of Child and Adolescent Psychiatry.*

Walrath, C. M., Nickerson, K. J., Crowel, R. L., & Leaf, P. J. (1998). Serving children with serious emotional disturbance in a system of care: Do mental health and non-mental health agency referrals look the same? *Journal of Emotional and Behavioral Disorders, 6,* 205–213.

Walrath, C. M., Sharp, M. J., Zuber, M., & Leaf, P. J. (2001). Serving children with SED in urban systems of care: Referral agency differences in child characteristics in Baltimore and the Bronx. *Journal of Emotional and Behavioral Disorders, 9,* 94–105.

Wolff, N. (2000). Using randomized trials to evaluate socially complex services: Problems, challenges and recommendations. *The Journal of Mental Health Policy and Economics, 3,* 97–109.

Wood, M., Chung, A., Furlong, M. J., Casas, J. M., Holbrook, L., & Richey, R. (1998). What works in a system of care? Services and outcomes associated with a juvenile probation population. *Journal of Juvenile Law and Policy, 2,* 63–71.

Wood, M., Furlong, M. J., Casas, J. M., & Sosna, T. (1998). A system of care for juvenile probationers. *Journal of Juvenile Law and Policy, 2,* 5–9.

Woodbridge, M., & Huang, L. (2000). Using evaluation data to manage, improve, market, and sustain children's services. *Systems of care: Promising practices in children's mental health, 2000 series, volume II.* Washington, DC: Center for Effective Collaboration and Practice, American Institutes for Research.

CHILDREN'S SERVICES: SOCIAL POLICY, RESEARCH, AND PRACTICE, 5(1), 67–74
Copyright © 2002, Lawrence Erlbaum Associates, Inc.

COMMENTARY

The National Evaluation of the Comprehensive Community Mental Health Services for Children and Their Families Program: A Commentary

Robert M. Friedman and Mario Hernandez
Department of Child and Family Studies
Louis de la Parte Florida Mental Health Institute
University of South Florida

In this article we comment on the other articles in this issue, which describe the national evaluation of the Comprehensive Community Mental Health Services for Children and Their Families Program. The commentary focuses on 4 major themes. The first theme is the complexity of community-based systems of care and the special challenge that this presents for their evaluation. The second theme is the need for theories of change for systems of care to be more clearly developed and elucidated. The third theme discusses the implications of the diversity of the population served for the development of interventions and for the application of interventions that have been tested on other populations. The fourth theme examines strategies for conducting evaluations, given the constraints that exist in large evaluations of community-wide interventions.

The Surgeon General of the United States has declared that "the burden of suffering experienced by children with mental health needs and their families has created a health crisis in this country" (Satcher, 2000, p. 1). Since the mid-1980s, the major approach within the public mental health system to addressing the needs of those

Requests for reprints should be sent to Robert M. Friedman, Department of Child and Family Studies, Louis de la Parte Florida Mental Health Institute, University of South Florida, 13301 Bruce B. Downs Boulevard, Tampa, FL 33612–3899. E-mail: friedman@hal.fmhi.usf.edu youngsters with the most serious emotional disturbances, and their families, has been through the development of community-based systems of care (Friedman, 2001; Holden, Friedman, & Santiago, 2001; Stroul, 1996; Stroul & Friedman, 1986). This special issue of *Children's Services: Social Policy, Research and Practice* takes a look at how well we are doing at developing such systems of care within the Comprehensive Community Mental Health Services for Children and Their Families Program, of the federal CMHS.

Rather than reviewing each of the articles in this special issue, this Commentary examines some general issues involved in developing and evaluating systems of care and discusses them in the context of the articles. The intent is both to comment on the articles and to advance the discussion about the development and evaluation of systems of care.

SYSTEMS OF CARE ARE HIGHLY COMPLEX, CREATING A MAJOR CHALLENGE FOR THEIR EVALUATION

Systems of care are neither specific nor simple interventions. Rather, when a community decides to implement a system of care, it is making a general statement of policy. It is indicating that it wants to establish a complex system targeted at a specific population of children and families, based on a widely agreed on set of principles and values and on the best available research (Stroul, 1996; Stroul & Friedman, 1986). The specific form that the system may take, however, can vary greatly.

One of the first tasks in evaluating a program or policy is determining how to describe it and measure it. Unless one can determine that the program or policy under study has been properly implemented, the results of an evaluation cannot be adequately interpreted. Given the complexity and variations in systems of care, this is a special challenge. It is particularly a challenge in a multisite evaluation, such as the evaluation of the federal CMHS program described in this special issue. The article in this issue by Brannan, Baughman, Reed, and Katz-Leavy (2002) describes how the evaluators went about measuring the degree to which a system of care was implemented in each community. This was done in two major domains. These are the infrastructure domain, which includes the organizational arrangements and procedures that are put into place to support actual service delivery, and the service delivery domain, which includes the activities and processes involved in delivering services and supports to children and families. This is a commendable effort, especially because the national evaluators had to develop this measurement approach at the same time as the grant program was being implemented nationally. Notwithstanding this commendable effort, however, the findings from this evaluation must be interpreted cautiously, given the preliminary stage of development of efforts to measure systems of care.

It is also noteworthy that systems of care are not static. They are constantly changing and evolving. As the article by Stroul, Pires, Armstrong, and Zaro (2002) indicates, this evaluation was undertaken at a time of rapid change in the financing of mental health services in many communities. Managed care procedures, which are implemented at least partially for cost control purposes, were instituted in many communities at the same time as these communities were receiving a new and sizeable federal grant, creating an additional challenge for the overall evaluation. Fortunately, the evaluators did not elect to ignore this important infrastructure change that was taking place. Rather, the evaluators decided to seize the opportunity to learn about the interaction between system of care development and the introduction of managed care financing procedures.

Another source of complexity lies in understanding the relation between the organizational–infrastructure level and the practice or service delivery level. How are organizational and infrastructure processes related to the services actually received and the outcomes achieved? Conversely, how do service practices and needs influence organizational and policy variables? These questions reflect an identified research question in the Surgeon General's Report on Mental Health (U.S. Department of Health and Human Services, 1999). That is, the need to better understand the relation between the organizational variables at the system level and variables at the practice level.

THE THEORY OF CHANGE FOR SYSTEMS OF CARE NEEDS FURTHER DEVELOPMENT

The conceptual framework for systems of care is designed to be a general model, allowing and encouraging flexibility and creativity in its application within communities. Largely due to the model's adaptable nature, policy makers, evaluators, researchers, and program staff must conceptualize and operationalize the model so that it can be implemented locally. This conceptualization of how the different pieces of the model will fit together to serve the population of concern and achieve the desired outcome can be called the "theory of change." Weiss (1995) pointed out that all social programs are based on a theory of how and why the program is expected to work, whether the theory is explicitly stated or not. It is suggested that programs that have well-articulated, explicit theories of change are more likely to be successful than those that do not (Hernandez & Hodges, 2001). Yet such theories of change are still in a relatively early stage of development, and many constructs, although generally described, have not been clearly defined. This includes such constructs as "individualized care," "cultural competence," and "collaboration."

The article by Manteuffel, Stephens, and Santiago (2002) includes an effort by the evaluators to describe the theory of change for systems of care. This is very helpful but the model that is presented, understandably, is still very general, and there are no indications that it has been adopted or adapted for use in many of the grant communities. So any multisite evaluation of systems of care must deal with the reality that different communities will be operating under different theories of change, in many cases the theories of change will not be explicit, the definition of key constructs within the theories is often vague, and the nature of the relation between different components of the system is unclear. The challenge to the children's mental health field is to do further work on the theory of change for purposes of advancing and strengthening system development efforts, as well as facilitating evaluation (Friedman, 1997).

THE POPULATION OF CHILDREN AND FAMILIES TO BE SERVED IS ENORMOUSLY DIVERSE

As indicated in the results presented by Manteuffel et al. (2002), and in other reviews of children served in public mental health systems (Friedman, Kutash, & Duchnowski, 1996; Liao, Manteuffel, Paulic, & Sondheimer, 2001), the children and adolescents served in local systems of care are diverse in age, gender, race, ethnicity, culture, diagnosis, co-occurring conditions, risk and protective factors, family constellation, and other characteristics. Part of this diversity can be attributed to the diversity of demonstration sites across the country. These sites represent inner city neighborhoods, midsize cities and counties, rural areas, Native American tribal organizations, and entire states. This indicates that one intended goal of systems of care, to reach a large and diverse population, has been achieved. It also makes the task of developing and implementing effective interventions very complex and challenging.

Although there has been a strong emphasis in recent years to implement interventions that have been rigorously tested and found to be effective, in most cases those interventions have not been tested on the populations of concern in systems of care, given the multiple and interrelated needs and strengths of this population. The diversity of the population served in systems of care stands in stark contrast to the populations of children studied in traditional clinical research, where, as Shirk (2001) pointed out, the emphasis has been on "the application of a well-defined treatment delivered by well-trained therapists to a set of children with well-demarcated problems" (p. 44). In fact, in reviewing findings from a task force of the American Psychological Association on empirically supported treatments, Weisz and Hawley (1998) indicated that "most of the treatments identified thus far … have been tested neither in conventional clinics nor under conditions that very much resemble applied clinical practice" (p. 212). Consequently, we actually know little about whether these treatments will be effective within operating systems of care serving diverse populations of children and adolescents. Weisz (2000) advocated for increased efforts at development of interventions in more naturalistic clinical settings rather than in special lab settings, and Burns (2000) pointed out that those interventions that have been shown to be effective with diverse populations, such as case management, therapeutic foster care, and multisystemic therapy, were actually developed in the field rather than in specialized clinic settings. Although it is encouraging that there are some interventions that have been developed and tested in the field and found to be effective, a major challenge to the children's mental health field is to expand the range of evidence-based interventions that have been shown to work with those youngsters and their families who are actually served in community settings (Friedman, 2000).

EVALUATION STRATEGIES MUST BE
SELECTED APPROPRIATELY

In determining the impact of an intervention, the "gold standard" in research and evaluation is the clinical trial in which participants are randomly assigned to two or more conditions, and everything is held constant except for the treatment of concern. Although this is possible in clinical research, in interventions that are community-wide this is in fact not possible. In discussing comprehensive community-wide initiatives, Hollister and Hill (1995) indicated that "community-wide programs present special problems for evaluators because the 'nectar of the gods'—random assignment of individuals to program treatment and to a control group—is beyond their reach" (p. 158).

This is a particular challenge in this service grant program, where demonstration sites have been selected in a nonrandom process based on of the merits of their application. In this evaluation, one effort to address this has been to identify, after the fact, communities that are similar to grant communities in as many ways as possible but do not have federally funded systems of care in place to serve as comparisons. Although such efforts to create post hoc comparison groups are problematic, particularly when the task requires identifying comparable communities, the results of such comparisons can still be a useful complement to other data collection efforts. Data collection for a large-scale comparison study has been completed within the national evaluation with a second-generation comparison study currently underway.

The fact that this grant program does not lend itself to a clean evaluation using a tight experimental design does not mean that there is not much to be learned. As the article by Holden, De Carolis, and Huff (2002) illustrates, this evaluation has used a broad knowledge development focus in an effort not only to determine the overall effectiveness of systems of care but to develop policy at the federal, state, and local level that serves children and families well. In discussing evaluation, Brown (1995) advocated an approach that places "less emphasis on discovering the one, objective truth about a program's worth and more attention to the multiple perspectives that diverse interests bring to judgment and understanding" (p. 204). Through the use of information from multiple sources, and through the use of a variety of quantitative and qualitative methodologies, the evaluators have sought to heed Brown's recommendation about overall knowledge development and recognized that there is much more to be learned than just an answer to the simplistic question of whether the program was effective.

In summary, this special issue includes four articles that describe different aspects of a very large and complex evaluation of a very large and complex initiative taking place in diverse communities around the country. The articles have done an excellent job of describing the theory of change for the initiative, describing the population to be served, developing a methodology to assess systems of care and capturing data on the development of such systems, examining the relation between systems of care and managed care, and using the findings to strengthen policy at all levels of government. The evaluation has used multiple methods and given voice to many different stakeholders in the process. The findings from the evaluation are likely to be important for assessing the current level of usefulness of systems of care in actualizing its principles of individualized, community-bound, and culturally competent care. However, the greatest value of the evaluation may be in stimulating improvements in the children's mental health field through questions it raises about such issues as the theory of change for systems of care, the precise meaning of some general constructs that are important within systems of care, the relation between the infrastructure level and the service delivery level, and the type of intervention development work that is needed to serve as diverse a population as that intended to be served.

ACKNOWLEDGMENTS

Work on this manuscript was supported by Contract Numbers 280–97–8014, 280–99–8023, and 280–00–8040 with the Child and Family Branch of the Center for Mental Health Services in the federal Substance Abuse and Mental Health Services Administration, United States Department of Health and Human Services.

REFERENCES

Brannan, A. M., Baughman, L. N., Reed, E. D., & Katz-Leavy, J. (2002/this issue). System-of-care assessment: Cross-site comparison of findings. *Children's Services: Social Policy, Research, and Practice, 5,* 37–56.

Brown, P. (1995). The role of the evaluator in comprehensive community initiatives. In J. P. Connell, A. C. Kubisch, L. B. Schorr, & C. H. Weiss (Eds.), *New approaches to evaluating community initiatives* (pp. 201–225). Washington, DC: Georgetown University Press.

Burns, B. B. (2000). Conference proceedings. In U.S. Public Health Service (Ed.), *Report of the Surgeon General's conference on children's mental health: A national action agenda* (pp. 35–36). Washington, DC: U.S. Public Health Service.

Friedman, R. M. (1997). Services and service delivery systems for children with serious emotional disorders: Issues in assessing effectiveness. In C. T. Nixon & D. A. Northrup (Eds.), *Evaluating mental health services: How do programs for children "work" in the real world?* (Vol. 3, pp. 16–43). Thousand Oaks, CA: Sage.

Friedman, R. M. (2000). Conference proceedings. In U.S. Public Health Service (Ed.), *Report of the Surgeon General's conference on children's mental health: A national action agenda* (pp. 43–44). Washington, DC: U.S. Public Health Service.

Friedman, R. M. (2001). The practice of psychology with children, adolescents, and their families: A look to the future. In J. N. Hughes, A. M. La Greca, & J. C. Conoley (Eds.), *Handbook of psychological services for children and adolescents* (pp. 3–22). New York: Oxford Press.

Friedman, R. M., Kutash, K., & Duchnowski, A. J. (1996). The population of concern: Defining the issues. In B. A. Stroul (Ed.), *Children's mental health: Creating systems of care in a changing society* (pp. 69–96). Baltimore: Brookes.

Hernandez, M., & Hodges, S. (2001). Using theory-based accountability to support systems of care. In M. Hernandez & S. Hodges (Eds.), *Tools, case studies and frameworks for developing outcome accountability in children's mental health.* Baltimore: Brookes.

Holden, E. W., De Carolis, G., & Huff, B. (2002/this issue). Policy implications of the national evaluation of the comprehensive community mental health services for children and their families program. *Children's Services: Social Policy, Research, and Practice, 5,* 57–65.

Holden, E. W., Friedman, R. M., & Santiago, R. L. (2001). Overview of the national evaluation of the comprehensive community mental health services for children and their families program. *Journal of Emotional and Behavioral Disorders, 9,* 4–12.

Hollister, R. G., & Hill, J. (1995). Problems in the evaluation of community-wide initiatives. In J. P. Connell, A. C. Kubisch, L. B. Schorr, & C. H. Weiss (Eds.), *New approaches to evaluating community initiatives: concepts, methods, and contexts* (pp. 127–172). Washington, DC: Aspen Institute.

Liao, Q., Manteuffel, B., Paulic, C., & Sondheimer, D. (2001). Describing the population of adolescents served in systems of care. *Journal of Emotional and Behavioral Disorders, 9,* 13–29.

Manteuffel, B., Stephens, R. L., & Santiago, R. (2002/this issue). Overview of the national evaluation of the comprehensive community mental health services for children and their families program and summary of current findings. *Children's Services: Social Policy, Research, and Practice, 5,* 3–20.

Satcher, D. (2000). Conference proceedings. In U.S. Public Health Service (Ed.), *Report of the Surgeon General's conference on children's mental health: A national action agenda* (pp. 17–18). Washington, DC: U.S. Public Health Service.

Shirk, S. R. (2001). The road to effective child psychological services: Treatment processes and outcome research. In J. N. Hughes, A. M. La Greca, & J. C. Conoley (Eds.), *Handbook of psychological services for children and adolescents* (pp. 43–59). New York: Oxford University Press.

Stroul, B. A. (1996). Children's mental health: Creating systems of care in a changing society. Baltimore: Brookes.

Stroul, B. A., & Friedman, R. M. (1986). *A system of care for children and youth with severe emotional disturbances* (Rev. ed.). Washington, DC: Georgetown University Child Development Center, CASSP Technical Assistance Center.

Stroul, B. A., Pires, S. A., Armstrong, M. I., & Zaro, S. (2002/this issue). The impact of managed care on systems of care that serve children with serious emotional disturbances and their families. *Children's Services: Social Policy, Research, and Practice, 5,* 21–36.

U.S. Department of Health and Human Services. (1999). *Mental Health: A Report of the Surgeon General.* Rockville, MD: U.S. Department of Health and Human Services, Substance Abuse and Mental

Health Services Administration, Center for Mental Health Services, National Institutes of Health, National Institute of Mental Health.

Weiss, C. H. (1995). Nothing as practical as good theory: Exploring theory-based evaluation for comprehensive community initiatives for children and families In J. P. Connell, A. C. Kubisch, L. B. Schorr, & C. H. Weiss (Eds.), *New approaches to evaluating community initiatives: concepts, methods, and contexts* (pp. 127–172). Washington, DC: Aspen Institute.

Weisz, J. R. (2000). Lab–clinic differences and what we can do about them. *Clinical Child Psychology Newsletter, 15,* 1–4.

Weisz, J. R., & Hawley, K. M. (1998). Finding, evaluating, refining, and applying empirically supported treatments for children and adolescents. *Journal of Clinical Child Psychology, 27,* 206–216.

For Product Safety Concerns and Information please contact our EU
representative GPSR@taylorandfrancis.com
Taylor & Francis Verlag GmbH, Kaufingerstraße 24, 80331 München, Germany

www.ingramcontent.com/pod-product-compliance
Ingram Content Group UK Ltd.
Pitfield, Milton Keynes, MK11 3LW, UK
UKHW020945180425
457613UK00019B/527